Student Workbook to Accompany Introduction to Medical Terminology

Ann Ehrlich
Carol L. Schroeder

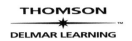

Student Workbook to Accompany Introduction to Medical Terminology
by Ann Ehrlich and Carol L. Schroeder

Executive Director:
William Brottmiller

Executive Editor:
Cathy L. Esperti

Acquisitions Editor:
Sherry Gomoll

Developmental Editor:
Deb Flis

Executive Marketing Manager:
Dawn F. Gerrain

Channel Manager:
Jennifer McAvey

Marketing Coordinator:
Mona Caron

Editorial Assistant:
Jennifer Conklin

Executive Production Manager:
Karen Leet

Art/Design Coordinator:
Robert Plante

Production Coordinator:
Catherine Ciardullo

Project Editor
David Buddle

Library of Congress Catalog Number 2002073641

ISBN-13: 978-1-4018-1140-2
ISBN-10: 1-4018-1140-X

Contents

Preface

TO THE STUDENT

Welcome to the *Student Workbook to Accompany Introduction to Medical Terminology*. This workbook contains many features to make your mastery of medical terminology easier, and it is to your benefit to take advantage of them.

CHAPTER ORGANIZATION

FLASH CARDS

The flash card pages at the back of this workbook are designed to be removed and used as flash cards. Flash cards are a great study aid, and early in your course you'll want to follow the instructions for removing these pages, separating the cards, and using them in a variety of fun study activities.

CHAPTER FEATURES

There is a chapter in this workbook to accompany each chapter in your textbook. Each workbook chapter includes the 100 Learning Exercises. To make these activities more interesting and challenging, they are in a variety of formats. With each question there is space for you to *write* your answer in the workbook. After you complete the exercises, follow your teacher's instructions for handing in your work and having it graded. When these pages are returned to you, save them in your notebook for use as an additional review resource.

Writing the answer to each question, rather than just circling a letter, reinforces the material you are learning. Many questions include a variety of answer choices and you'll be pleasantly surprised at how quickly you can complete the exercises!

WORD PART REVIEW

There is a Word Part Review section to be completed after you have studied chapters 1 and 2. This short section provides additional practice in working with word parts ,plus a test to evaluate how well you've mastered their use.

Because most medical terms are based on word parts, mastery of these component's is very importnant before you begin your study of the body systems. If you have trouble here, this is time to ask for help!

COMPREHENSIVE REVIEW

At the end of your workbook there is a Comprehensive Medical Terminology Review section. This contains Study Tips, Review Questions, and a simulated Final Test all of which are designed to help you prepare for the final examination. You'll find this section very helpful when you use it on your own or in conjunction with class review sessions.

GOOD LUCK!

It is our hope that your study of medical terminology will be interesting and rewarding. We also hope that this text and workbook help you find a career in health care that will bring you professional success and satisfaction.

Carol Schroeder
Ann Ehrlich

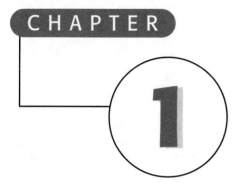

CHAPTER 1

Introduction to Medical Terminology

LEARNING EXERCISES

Grade _____ Name _____

MATCHING WORD PARTS 1

Write the correct answer in the middle column.

Definition	Correct Answer	Possible Answers
1.1. bad, difficult, painful	_____	-algia
1.2. excessive, increased	_____	dys-
1.3. liver	_____	-ectomy
1.4. pain, suffering	_____	hepat/o
1.5. surgical removal	_____	hyper-

MATCHING WORD PARTS 2

Write the correct answer in the middle column.

Definition	Correct Answer	Possible Answers
1.6. abnormal condition	_____	hypo-
1.7. abnormal softening	_____	-itis
1.8. deficient, decreased	_____	-malacia
1.9. inflammation	_____	-necrosis
1.10. tissue death	_____	-osis

MATCHING WORD PARTS 3

Write the correct answer in the middle column.

Definition	Correct Answer	Possible Answers
1.11. bleeding	_____	-ostomy
1.12. surgical creation of an opening	_____	-otomy
1.13. surgical incision	_____	-plasty
1.14. surgical repair	_____	-rrhage
1.15. to suture	_____	-rrhaphy

MATCHING WORD PARTS 4

Write the correct answer in the middle column.

Definition	Correct Answer	Possible Answers
1.16. visual examination	_____	-rrhea
1.17. rupture	_____	-rrhexis
1.18. abnormal narrowing	_____	-sclerosis
1.19. abnormal hardening	_____	-scopy
1.20. abnormal flow	_____	-stenosis

DEFINITIONS

Select the correct answer and write it on the line provided.

1.21. The word part meaning plaque or fatty substance is _____.

    -algia   arteri/o   ather/o   arthr/o

1.22. The prefix meaning surrounding is _____.

    inter-   intra-   peri-   pre-

1.23. A _____ is always placed at the end of the term.

    combining form   prefix   suffix   word root

1.24. The word part meaning white is _____.

    cyan/o   erythr/o   leuk/o   poli/o

1.25. The suffix meaning abnormal softening is _____.

    -malacia   -necrosis   -sclerosis   -stenosis

1.26. Pain, which can be observed only by the patient, is a _____.

    prognosis   remission   sign   symptom

1.27. The prefix meaning deficient or decreased is _____.

    hyper-   hypo-   peri-   supra-

1.28. A _____ is a prediction of the probable course and outcome of a disease.

diagnose   diagnosis   prognosis   syndrome

1.29. The suffix meaning to rupture is _____.

-rrhage   -rrhaphy   -rrhea   -rrhexis

1.30. The plural of the term appendix is _____.

appendexes   appendices   appendixes   appendizes

MATCHING TERMS AND DEFINITIONS

Write the correct answer in the middle column.

Definition	Correct Answer	Possible Answers
1.31. examination procedure	_____	laceration
1.32. male gland	_____	lesion
1.33. pathologic tissue change	_____	palpitation
1.34. pounding heart	_____	palpation
1.35. torn, ragged wound	_____	prostate

WHICH WORD?

Select the correct answer and write it on the line provided.

1.36. The body cavities are lined with specialized _____ membrane.

mucous   mucus

1.37. The formation of pus is called _____.

supination   suppuration

1.38. The term meaning wound or injury is _____.

trauma   triage

1.39. The term meaning possessing masculine traits is _____.

    viral   virile

1.40. The term describing part of the small intestine is _____.

    ileum   ilium

SPELLING COUNTS

Find the misspelled word in each sentence. Then write that word, spelled correctly, on the line provided.

1.41. A disease named for the person who discovered it is known as an enaponym. _____

1.42. A localized response to injury or tissue destruction is called inflimmation.

_____

1.43. The act of closing a wound by stitching is sutering. _____

1.44. The medical term meaning the surgical repair of a nerve is neuriplasty. _____

1.45. The medical term meaning inflammation of the tonsils is tonsilitis. _____

MATCHING TERMS

Write the correct answer in the middle column.

Definition	Correct Answer	Possible Answers
1.46. abnormal stomach condition	_____	cardiac
1.47. pertaining to the heart	_____	gastralgia
1.48. rupture of a muscle	_____	gastrosis
1.49. stomach pain	_____	myoplasty
1.50. surgical muscle repair	_____	myorrhexis

TERM SELECTION

Select the correct answer and write it on the line provided.

1.51. The abnormal narrowing of an artery or arteries is called _____.

arteriosclerosis   arteriostenosis   arthrostenosis   atherosclerosis

1.52. Based on the word part that indicates color, the term _____ means blue skin coloration due to the lack of oxygen.

cyanosis   erythrocytes   leukocytes   melanosis

1.53. The term _____ contains a combining vowel between two word roots.

abdominocentesis   endoscopy   gastroenteritis   hemorrhage

1.54. The prefix _____ means bad, difficult, or painful.

-algia   -dynia   dys-   eu-

1.55. A _____ is a specialist in diagnosing and treating diseases, disorders, and problems associated with aging.

gerontologist   gerontology   neurologist   neurology

SENTENCE COMPLETION

Write the correct term on the line provided.

1.56. Lower than normal blood pressure is called _____.

1.57. The process of recording a picture of an artery or arteries is called _____.

1.58. The term meaning above or outside the ribs is _____.

1.59. A strong dependence on a drug or substance is known as a/an _____.

1.60. The act of binding or tying off blood vessels or ducts is called _____.

TRUE/FALSE

If the statement is true, write **T** on the line. If the statement is false, write **F** on the line.

1.61. _____ Arterionecrosis is the abnormal narrowing of an artery or arteries.

1.62. _____ Mucus is the substance secreted by the mucous membranes.

1.63. _____ Supination is the formation or discharging of pus.

1.64. _____ A suffix usually, but not always, indicates location, time, or number.

1.65. _____ A combining vowel is used when the suffix begins with a consonant.

1.66. _____ Ova is the plural of ovum.

1.67. _____ A disease that is in remission has been cured.

1.68. _____ The term phlegm begins with an F sound.

1.69. _____ To diagnose is the process of reaching a diagnosis.

1.70. _____ It is not necessary to use a combining vowel when joining two root words.

CLINICAL CONDITIONS

Write the correct answer on the line provided.

1.71. Beverly Gaston suffers from higher than normal blood pressure. This is recorded on her chart as

_____.

1.72. Mrs. Tillson was treated for pulmonary _____. This condition is an excessive

buildup of fluid in the lungs.

1.73. Dr. Gusterson is trained in the treatment of the diseases and disorders associated with aging. His specialty is

known as _____.

1.74. In an accident, Felipe Valladares suffered a broken toe. The medical term for this is a fractured

_____.

1.75. Hal Jamison received emergency treatment for _____, which is an inflamma-

tion of the appendix.

1.76. Gina Manley told her friends that she has an enlarged liver. The medical term for this condition is

_____.

1.77. As she used her hands to examine the patient, Dr. Liu was using an examination technique called

_____.

1.78. Joan Randolph's medication was administered by an injection into the muscle. This is called an

_____ or IM injection.

1.79. Andy Lewis describes that uncomfortable feeling as heartburn. The medical term for this condition is

_____.

1.80. Max Greene's muscle wound required suturing. This procedure is called _____.

WHICH IS THE CORRECT MEDICAL TERM?

Select the correct answer and write it on the line provided.

1.81. The term _____ means an inflammation of a nerve or nerves.

neuralgia   neuritis   neurology   neuroplasty

1.82. The term _____ means loss of a large amount of blood in a short time.

diarrhea   hemorrhage   hepatorrhagia   otorrhagia

1.83. The term _____ means the tissue death of an artery or arteries.

arteriomalacia   arterionecrosis   arteriosclerosis   arteriostenosis

1.84. The term _____ describes the time and events before birth.

neonatal   perinatal   postnatal   prenatal

1.85. The term _____ means enlargement of the liver.

hepatitis   hepatomegaly   nephromegaly   nephritis

CHALLENGE WORD BUILDING

These terms are not found in this chapter; however, they are made up of the following word parts. You may want to look in the textbook glossary or use a medical dictionary to check your answers.

neo- = new

arteri/o = artery

arthr/o = joint

cardi/o = heart

nat/o = birth

neur/o = nerve

rhin/o = nose

-algia = pain and suffering

-itis = inflammation

-ologist = specialist

-otomy = a surgical incision

-rrhea = abnormal flow

-scopy = visual examination

1.86. A medical specialist concerned with the diagnosis and treatment of heart disease is a/an

_____.

1.87. The term meaning a runny nose is _____.

1.88. The term meaning the inflammation of a joint is _____.

1.89. A specialist in disorders of the newborn is called a/an _____.

1.90. The term meaning a surgical incision into a nerve is a/an _____.

1.91. The term meaning the visual examination of the internal structure of a joint is

_____.

1.92. The term meaning an inflammation of an artery is _____.

1.93. The term meaning pain in a nerve or nerves is _____.

1.94. The term meaning a surgical incision into the heart is a/an _____.

1.95. The term meaning an inflammation of the nose is _____.

LABELING EXERCISES

Identify the numbered items in the accompanying figure.

1.96. The word part (combining form) meaning spinal cord is _____/_.

1.97. The word part (combining form) meaning muscle is _____/_.

1.98. The word part (combining form) meaning bone marrow is _____/_.

1.99. The word part (combining form) meaning nerve is _____/_.

1.100. The word part (combining form) meaning joint is _____/_.

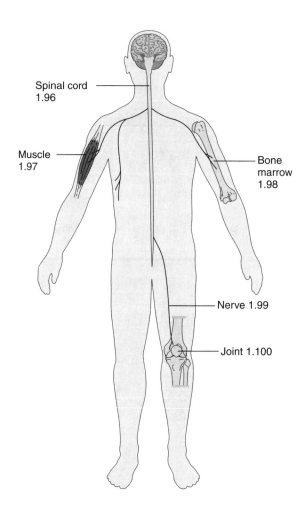

Spinal cord 1.96

Muscle 1.97

Bone marrow 1.98

Nerve 1.99

Joint 1.100

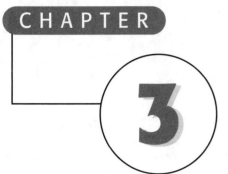

The Skeletal System

LEARNING EXERCISES

Grade _____ Name _____

MATCHING WORD PARTS 1

Write the correct answer in the middle column.

Definition	Correct Answer	Possible Answers
3.1. hump	_____	ankly/o
3.2. cartilage	_____	arthr/o
3.3. crooked, bent, or stiff	_____	-um
3.4. joint	_____	kyph/o
3.5. noun ending	_____	chondr/o

MATCHING WORD PARTS 2

Write the correct answer in the middle column.

Definition	Correct Answer	Possible Answers
3.6. cranium, skull	_____	cost/o
3.7. rib	_____	crani/o
3.8. setting free, loosening	_____	-desis
3.9. spinal cord, bone marrow	_____	-lysis
3.10. surgical fixation of bone or joint	_____	myel/o

MATCHING WORD PARTS 3

Write the correct answer in the middle column.

Definition	Correct Answer	Possible Answers
3.11. vertebra, vertebral column	_____	oste/o
3.12. curved	_____	spondyl/o
3.13. bent backward	_____	lord/o
3.14. pertaining to formation	_____	-poietic
3.15. bone	_____	scolio

DEFINITIONS

Select the correct answer and write it on the line provided.

3.16. The term that describes the shaft of a long bone is _____.

    diaphysis   distal epiphysis   endosteum   proximal epiphysis

3.17. The tarsals are the bones that make up the _____.

    ankles   fingers   toes   wrist

3.18. The upper portion of the sternum is the _____.

    clavicle   mandible   manubrium   xiphoid process

3.19. The _____ joints are movable.

    cartilaginous   fibrous   suture   synovial

3.20. The anterior portion of the pelvic girdle is known as the _____.

    ilium   ischium   pubis   sacrum

3.21. The blood vessels, nerves, and ligaments pass through an opening in a bone known as a

    _____.

    fontanel   foramen   meatus   suture

3.22. The tissue that connects one bone to another bone is known as a/an _____.

    articular cartilage   ligament   synovial membrane   tendon

3.23. The hip socket is known as the _____.

    acetabulum   malleolus   patella   trochanter

3.24. The bones of the fingers and toes are called _____.

    carpals   metatarsals   tarsals   phalanges

3.25. A normal projection on the surface of a bone is a/an _____.

    cruciate   exostosis   popliteal   process

MATCHING STRUCTURES

Write the correct answer in the middle column.

Definition	Correct Answer	Possible Answers
3.26. breastbone	_____	clavicle
3.27. cheek bone	_____	olecranon
3.28. collar bone	_____	sternum
3.29. kneecap	_____	patella
3.30. point of the elbow	_____	zygomatic

WHICH WORD?

Select the correct answer and write it on the line provided.

3.31. The surgical procedure to loosen an ankylosed joint is called _____.

    arthrodesis   arthrolysis

3.32. A physician who specializes in the diagnosis and treatment of diseases characterized by inflammation in the connective tissues is a/an _____.

    orthopedist   rheumatologist

3.33. An _____ transplant uses bone marrow from a donor.

    allogenic   autologous

3.34. The term meaning the surgical repair of the skull is a _____.

    craniectomy   cranioplasty

3.35. The type of arthritis that is commonly known as wear-and-tear arthritis is _____.

    osteoarthritis   rheumatoid arthritis

SPELLING COUNTS

Find the misspelled word in each sentence. Then write that word, spelled correctly, on the line provided.

3.36. The medical term for the condition commonly known as low back pain is lumbaego.

_____

3.37. Ostealgea means any pain that is linked to an abnormal condition with a bone.

_____

3.38. Ankylosing spondilitis is an inflammatory joint disease characterized by progressive stiffening of the spine caused by fusion of the vertebral bodies.

_____

3.39. The term meaning suturing or wiring together of bones is osterrhaphy.

_____

3.40. The sound heard when the ends of a broken bone move together is called crepetation.

_____

MATCHING TERMS AND DEFINITIONS

Write the correct answer in the middle column.

Definition	Correct Answer	Possible Answers
3.41. closed reduction	_____	closed fracture
3.42. clubfoot	_____	manipulation
3.43. compound fracture	_____	open fracture
3.44. osteitis deformans	_____	Paget's disease
3.45. simple fracture	_____	talipes

TERM SELECTION

Select the correct answer and write it on the line provided.

3.46. The term meaning the death of bone tissue is _____.

osteitis deformans   osteomyelitis   osteonecrosis   osteoporosis

3.47. An abnormal increase in the forward curvature of the lower or lumbar spine is known as

_____.

kyphosis   lordosis   scoliosis   spondylosis

3.48. The condition known as _____ is a congenital defect.

juvenile arthritis   osteoarthritis   rheumatoid arthritis   spina bifida

3.49. A malignant tumor composed of cells derived from blood-forming tissues of the bone marrow is known as

a/an _____.

chondroma   Ewing's sarcoma   myeloma   osteochondroma

3.50. The bulging deposit that forms around the area of the break during the healing of a fractured bone is a

_____.

callus   crepitation   crepitus   luxation

SENTENCE COMPLETION

Write the correct term on the line provided.

3.51. The general term used to describe a variety of acute and chronic conditions characterized by inflammation and deterioration of connective tissues is _____.

3.52. The partial displacement of a bone from its joint is known as _____.

3.53. The medical term for the procedure also known as fusion, that stiffens a joint or joining of several vertebrae, is _____.

3.54. The medical term for the surgical removal of a spinal lamina is a/an _____.

3.55. A hallux valgus is commonly known as a/an _____.

TRUE/FALSE

If the statement is true, write **T** on the line. If the statement is false, write **F** on the line.

3.56. _____ A percutaneous diskectomy is performed through the skin of the back.

3.57. _____ A craniotomy is a surgical incision into the collar bone.

3.58. _____ Spondylolisthesis is a subluxation of one vertebra over the one below it.

3.59. _____ Osteoclasis is a pathologic condition that involves abnormal hardening of the bones.

3.60. _____ Arthrocentesis is the surgical removal of fluid from a joint.

3.61. _____ When a bone is broken at an angle, it is said to be an oblique fracture.

3.62. _____ Paget's disease is caused by a deficiency of calcium and vitamin D in early childhood.

3.63. _____ Stiffness of the joints, especially in the aged, is known as atherosclerosis.

3.64. _____ The loss or absence of mobility in a joint because the bones have abnormally fused together is known as ankylosis.

3.65. _____ The surgical removal of a bursa is a bursitis.

CLINICAL CONDITIONS

Write the correct answer on the line provided.

3.66. When Bobby Kuhn fell out of a tree, the bone in his arm was partially bent and partially broken. Dr. Parker described this as _____ fracture and told the family that this type of fracture occurs primarily in children.

3.67. Eduardo Sanchez has an inflammation of the bone and bone marrow. The medical term for this condition is _____.

3.68. Brent Hargraves, who is 16, was diagnosed as having _____ sarcoma. This is a group of cancers that most frequently affect children or adolescents.

3.69. Mrs. Morton suffers from dowager's hump. This medical term for this abnormal curvature of the spine is _____.

3.70. Henry Turner specializes in creating _____. These are orthopedic appliances to align, prevent, or correct deformities or to improve the function of movable parts of the body.

3.71. After an auto accident, Tiffany required _____ to repair the damage to her skull.

3.72. Mrs. Gilmer, who is 84 years old, fell and broke her hip. Her doctor repaired this fracture by placing pins to hold the bone together as it heals. These pins, which will not be removed, are known as _____ fixation.

3.73. Betty Greene has been running for several years; however, now her knees hurt. Dr. Baskin diagnosed that she has _____. This is an abnormal softening of the cartilage in these joints.

3.74. Patty Turner (age 7) has symptoms that include a skin rash, fever, slowed growth, fatigue, and swelling in the joints. She was diagnosed as having juvenile _____ arthritis.

3.75. Robert Young has a very sore shoulder. Dr. Wilson diagnosed it as an inflammation of the bursa and called it _____.

WHICH IS THE CORRECT MEDICAL TERM?

Select the correct answer and write it on the line provided.

3.76. Rodney Horner is being treated for a _____ fracture in which the ends of the bones were crushed together.

    Colles'   comminuted   compound   spiral

3.77. Alex Jordon's doctor performed a/an _____ to surgically repair the cartilage that Alex damaged when she fell.

    arthroplasty   chondritis   chondroplasty   osteoplasty

3.78. Jane Parker was concerned about bone loss after menopause. To evaluate her condition, Jane's doctor ordered a/an _____ test.

    bone scan   blood calcium   DXA   MRI

3.79. In an effort to return a fractured bone to normal alignment, Dr. Wong ordered _____. This procedure exerts a pulling force on the distal end of the affected limb.

    external fixation   immobilization   internal fixation   traction

3.80. Juanita was treated for an inflammation of the tissue surrounding a bone. This condition is known as

    _____.

    ostealgia   osteitis   osteomyelitis   periostitis

CHALLENGE WORD BUILDING

These terms are not found in this chapter; however, they are made up of the following familiar word parts. You may want to look in the textbook glossary or use a medical dictionary to check your answers.

poly-	arthr/o	-ectomy
	chondr/o	-itis
	cost/o	-malacia
	crani/o	-otomy
	oste/o	-pathy
		-sclerosis

3.81. Abnormal hardening of bone is called _____.

3.82. The surgical removal of a rib is a/an _____.

3.83. The term meaning a disease of the cartilage is _____.

3.84. A surgical incision into a joint is a/an _____.

3.85. The term meaning inflammation of cartilage is _____.

3.86. The surgical removal of a joint is a/an _____.

3.87. The term meaning inflammation of more than one joint is _____.

3.88. The term meaning any disease involving the bones and joints is _____.

3.89. A surgical incision or division of a rib is a/an _____.

3.90. The term meaning abnormal softening of the skull is _____.

LABELING EXERCISES

Identify the numbered items on the accompanying figures.

3.91. _____ vertebrae

3.92. _____

3.93. _____

3.94. _____

3.95. _____

3.96. _____

3.97. _____

3.98. _____

3.99. _____

3.100. _____

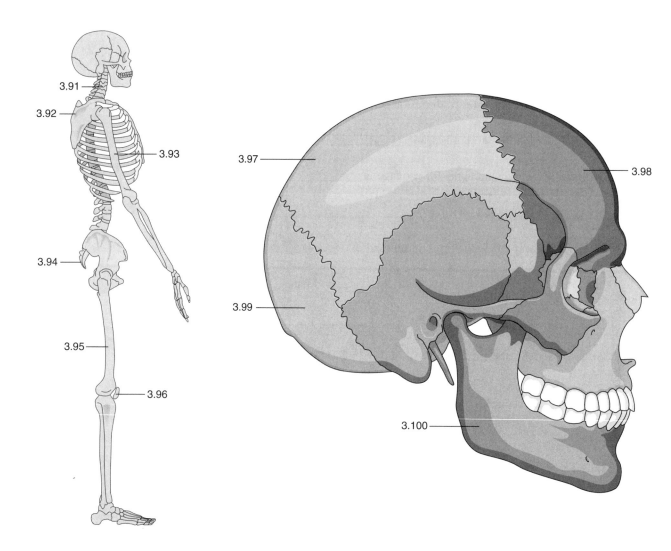

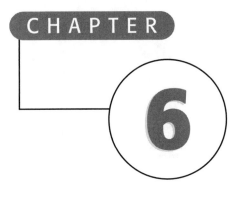

LEARNING EXERCISES

Grade _____ Name _____

MATCHING WORD PARTS 1

Write the correct answer in the middle column.

Definition	Correct Answer	Possible Answers
6.1. to destroy	_____	blast/o
6.2. neck	_____	carcin/o
6.3. eat, swallow	_____	cervic/o
6.4. cancer	_____	phag/o
6.5. immature, embryonic	_____	-lytic

MATCHING WORD PARTS 2

Write the correct answer in the middle column.

Definition	Correct Answer	Possible Answers
6.6. formation	_____	immun/o
6.7. flesh	_____	onc/o
6.8. protected, safe	_____	-plasm
6.9. spleen	_____	sarc/o
6.10. tumor	_____	splen/o

MATCHING TYPES OF PATHOGENS

Write the correct answer in the middle column.

Definition	Correct Answer	Possible Answers
6.11. bacteria capable of movement	_____	parasite
6.12. chain-forming bacteria	_____	spirochete
6.13. cluster-forming bacteria	_____	staphylococci
6.14. live only by invading cells	_____	streptococci
6.15. lives within another organism	_____	viruses

DEFINITIONS

Select the correct answer and write it on the line provided.

6.16. The structure(s) with a hemolytic function is/are the _____.

adenoids   lymph nodes   spleen   tonsils

6.17. The term meaning inflammation of the lymph nodes is _____.

adenoiditis   lymphadenitis   lymphedema   lymphoma

6.18. Herpes zoster is commonly known as _____.

3-day measles   chickenpox   German measles   shingles

6.19. The substance that causes noninfected cells to form an antiviral protein is called

_____.

complement   immunoglobulin   interferon   vaccine

6.20. The structure, composed largely of lymphatic tissue, that plays important roles in the immune and endocrine
systems is the _____.

bone marrow   liver   spleen   thymus

6.21. The structures that form a protective ring of lymphatic tissue surrounding the internal openings of the nose
and mouth are the _____.

adenoids   lacteals   lymph nodes   tonsils

6.22. Lymph vessels return intercellular fluid to the _____.

arteries   capillaries   cells   veins

6.23. The lacteals are located in the _____.

armpits   groin   neck   small intestine

6.24. The disease _____ is caused by a fungus.

aspergillosis   herpes zoster   malaria   Lyme disease

6.25. The type of cell that protects the body by eating invading cells is a _____.

B lymphocyte   lymphokine   macrophage   T lymphocyte

MATCHING STRUCTURES

Write the correct answer in the middle column.

Definition	Correct Answer	Possible Answers
6.26. acts as a physical barrier	_____	lymph nodes
6.27. filter harmful substances from lymph	_____	skin
6.28. has roles in lymphatic and endocrine systems	_____	spleen
6.29. lymphatic tissue hanging from the lower portion of the cecum	_____	thymus
6.30. stores extra erythrocytes	_____	vermiform appendix

WHICH WORD?

Select the correct answer and write it on the line provided.

6.31. The _____ direct the immune response by signaling between the cells of the immune system.

    lymphokines   macrophages

6.32. The growth of neoplasms is blocked by a/an _____ drug.

    antineoplastic   cytotoxic

6.33. Plasma cells develop from transformed _____.

    B cells   T cells

6.34. Hepatitis B and C may be treated using _____ that was created in the laboratory.

    immunoglobulin   interferon

6.35. Infectious mononucleosis is a _____ infection.

    bacterial   viral

SPELLING COUNTS

Find the misspelled word in each sentence. Then write that word, spelled correctly, on the line provided.

6.36. A sarkoma is a malignant tumor that arises from connective tissue. _____

6.37. The nasopharyngeal tonsils are also known as the adenods. _____

6.38. Reubella is also known as 3-day measles. _____

6.39. Antiobiotics are used to combat bacterial infections. _____

6.40. The condition commonly known as chickenpox is caused by the herpes virus Varicella soster.

_____

MATCHING ABBREVIATIONS

Write the correct answer in the middle column.

Definition	Correct Answer	Possible Answers
6.41. invasive ductal carcinoma	_____	Ca
6.42. Kaposi's sarcoma	_____	HL
6.43. invasive lobular carcinoma	_____	IDC
6.44. carcinoma	_____	ILC
6.45. Hodgkin's lymphoma	_____	KS

TERM SELECTION

Select the correct answer and write it on the line provided.

6.46. The term meaning not recurring and with a favorable chance for recovery is

_____.

    benign   in situ   malignant   neoplasm

6.47. The condition that is frequently associated with an HIV infection is _____.

    lymphoma   Hodgkin's disease   Kaposi's sarcoma   myoma

6.48. Malaria is caused by a _____.

   parasite   rickettsiae   spirochete   virus

6.49. An example of a disease caused by a bacillus is _____.

   aspergillosis   Lyme disease   rubella   tuberculosis

6.50. Koplik's spots in the mouth are an early sign of _____.

   measles   mumps   shingles   rubella

SENTENCE COMPLETION

Write the correct term on the line provided.

6.51. The term that describes a serious system allergic reaction, in which the patient can die within minutes, is

   _____.

6.52. In _____, radioactive materials are implanted into the tissues to be treated.

6.53. The _____ blot test is used to confirm a seropositive ELISA test for HIV.

6.54. A/An _____ is a benign abnormal collection of lymphatic vessels forming a mass.

6.55. Persistent generalized _____ is the continued presence of diffuse enlargement of lymph nodes.

TRUE/FALSE

If the statement is true, write **T** on the line. If the statement is false, write **F** on the line.

6.56. _____ Lymph fluid always flows toward the thoracic cavity.

6.57. _____ Splenomegaly means abnormal softening of the spleen.

6.58. _____ Lymphedema is an abnormal accumulation of fluid primarily in the legs and ankles.

6.59. _____ Acquired immunity is passed from the mother to child after birth.

6.60. _____ Reed-Sternberg cells are present in non-Hodgkin's lymphoma.

6.61. _____ Ductal carcinoma in situ accounts for the majority of all breast cancers.

6.62. _____ Teletherapy uses 3-dimensional computer imaging to aim radiation doses more precisely.

6.63. _____ Hodgkin's disease at stage I has a better cure rate than at stage IV.

6.64. _____ An osteosarcoma usually involves the bones of the sacrum.

6.65. _____ Breast cancer cannot occur in males because they do not have breast tissue.

CLINICAL CONDITIONS

Write the correct answer on the line provided.

6.66. Dr. Wei diagnosed her patient as having an enlarged spleen. The medical term for this condition is

_____.

6.67. The cause of Roger Thompson's infection was the _____. This is caused by a
group of large herpes-type viruses with a wide variety of disease effects.

6.68. Mr. Grossman was treated with a _____ drug. This is a hormone-like preparation used primarily as an anti-inflammatory and as an immunosuppressant.

6.69. Soon after her breast cancer was diagnosed, Dorothy Peterson's doctor performed a/an
_____. In this procedure the tumor and a margin of healthy tissue are removed.

6.70. Since his kidney transplant, Mr. Lanning must take a/an _____ to prevent
rejection of the donor organ.

6.71. José Sanchez received a poliomyelitis _____ to ensure his immunity to this
disease.

6.72. Tarana Inglis complained that the glands in her neck were swollen. Dr. Neilson explained that these are the
_____ lymph nodes.

6.73. Because he had chickenpox as a child, Rob Harris now has natural _____
immunity to this disease.

6.74. As a child, John Fogelman had a viral disease in which the parotid glands were swollen. John's doctor said
he had the _____.

6.75. Jane Doe is infected with HIV. One of her medications is acyclovir, which is a/an
_____ drug.

WHICH IS THE CORRECT MEDICAL TERM?

Select the correct answer and write it on the line provided.

6.76. The yeast Candida albicans causes _____.

aspergillus   chickenpox   moniliasis   rubella

6.77. Of the diseases listed here, _____ is the only one that is *not* an autoimmune disorder.

Crohn's disease   Graves' disease   lymphedema   psoriasis

6.78. The type of bacteria that are capable of movement are the _____.

bacilli   spirochetes   staphylococcus   streptococcus

6.79. An example of a soft tissue sarcoma is _____.

adenocarcinoma   myosarcoma   neurosarcoma   osteosarcoma

6.80. Endocarditis and pneumonia are usually caused by _____ infections.

fungal   staphylococci   streptococci   virus

CHALLENGE WORD BUILDING

These terms are *not* found in this chapter; however, they are made up of the following familiar word parts. You may want to look in the textbook glossary or use a medical dictionary to check your answers.

adenoid/o   -ectomy

immun/o   -itis

lymphaden/o   -ology

lymphang/o   -oma

splen/o   -rrhaphy

tonsill/o

thym/o

6.81. The study of the immune system is known as _____.

6.82. The term meaning surgical removal of the spleen is a/an _____.

6.83. The term meaning an inflammation of the thymus is _____.

6.84. The term meaning an inflammation of the lymph vessels is _____.

6.85. The term meaning to suture the spleen is _____.

6.86. The term meaning the surgical removal of the adenoids is a/an _____.

6.87. The term meaning the surgical removal of a lymph node is a/an _____.

6.88. The term meaning a tumor originating in the thymus is _____.

6.89. The term meaning an inflammation of the tonsils is _____.

6.90. The term meaning an inflammation of the spleen is _____.

LABELING EXERCISES

Identify the numbered items on the accompanying figures.

6.91. tonsils and _____

6.92. bone _____

6.93. appendix and _____

6.94. _____

6.95. _____

6.96. _____ lymphatic duct

6.97. _____ lymph nodes

6.98. _____ duct

6.99. _____ lymph nodes

6.100. _____ lymph nodes

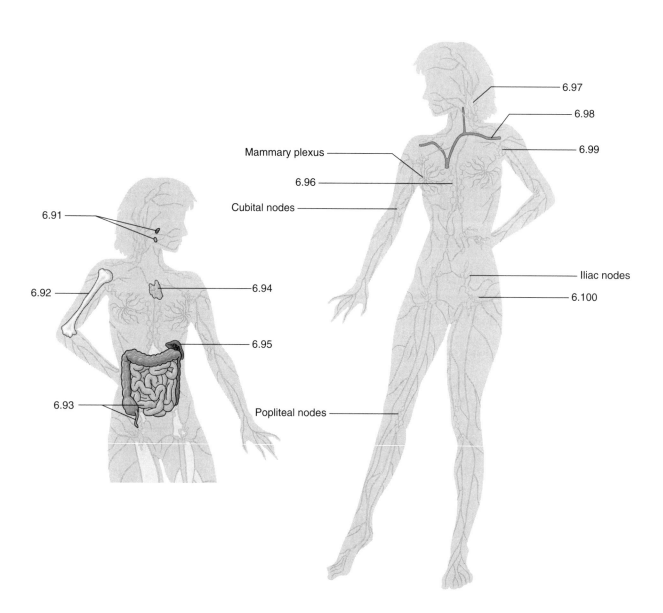

The Respiratory System

LEARNING EXERCISES

Grade _____ Name _____

MATCHING WORD PARTS 1

Write the correct answer in the middle column.

Definition	Correct Answer	Possible Answers
7.1. enlargement	_____	atel/o
7.2. voice box	_____	bronch/o
7.3. windpipe	_____	cyan/o
7.4. blue	_____	-ectasis
7.5. incomplete	_____	laryng/o

MATCHING WORD PARTS 2

Write the correct answer in the middle column.

Definition	Correct Answer	Possible Answers
7.6. lung	_____	ox/o
7.7. oxygen	_____	pharyng/o
7.8. multilayered membrane	_____	phon/o
7.9. throat	_____	pleur/o
7.10. voice	_____	pneum/o

MATCHING WORD PARTS 3

Write the correct answer in the middle column.

Definition	Correct Answer	Possible Answers
7.11. windpipe	_____	-pnea
7.12. rapid	_____	pulmon/o
7.13. lung	_____	tachy-
7.14. chest	_____	-thorax
7.15. breathing	_____	trache/o

DEFINITIONS

Select the correct answer and write it on the line provided.

7.16. The heart, aorta, esophagus, and trachea are located in the _____.

dorsal cavity   manubrium   mediastinum   pleura

7.17. The _____ acts as a lid over the entrance to esophagus.

Adam's apple   epiglottis   glottis   thyroid cartilage

Name _____

7.18. The innermost layer of the pleura is known as the _____.

parietal pleura   pleural space   plural cavity   visceral pleura

7.19. The _____ sinuses are located just above the eyes.

ethmoid   frontal   maxillary   sphenoid

7.20. The smallest divisions of the bronchial tree are the _____.

alveoli   alveolus   bronchioles   bronchi

7.21. During respiration, the exchange of gases takes place through the walls of the

_____.

alveoli   arteries   capillaries   veins

7.22. The term meaning spitting blood or blood-stained sputum is _____.

effusion   epistaxis   hemoptysis   hemothorax

7.23. Grinder's disease is the lay term for _____.

anthracosis   byssinosis   pneumoconiosis   silicosis

7.24. The term _____ means an abnormally rapid rate of respiration.

apnea   bradypnea   dyspnea   tachypnea

7.25. The term meaning any voice impairment is _____.

aphonia   dysphonia   laryngitis   laryngoplegia

MATCHING STRUCTURES

Write the correct answer in the middle column.

Definition	Correct Answer	Possible Answers
7.26. first division of the pharynx	_____	laryngopharynx
7.27. second division of the pharynx	_____	larynx
7.28. third division of the pharynx	_____	nasopharynx
7.29. voice box	_____	oropharynx
7.30. windpipe	_____	trachea

WHICH WORD?

Select the correct answer and write it on the line provided.

7.31. The exchange of gases within the cells of the body is known as _____ respiration.

    external   internal

7.32. The term that describes the lung disease caused by cotton, flax, or hemp dust is

    _____.

    anthracosis   byssinosis

7.33. The form of pneumonia that can be prevented through vaccination is _____ pneumonia.

    bacterial   viral

7.34. The term commonly known as shortness of breath is _____.

    dyspnea   eupnea

7.35. The emergency procedure to gain access below a blocked airway is called a

    _____.

    tracheostomy   tracheotomy

SPELLING COUNTS

Find the misspelled word in each sentence. Then write the word, spelled correctly, on the line provided.

7.36. The thick mucus secreted by the tissues that line the respiratory passages is called phlem.

    _____

7.37. The medical term meaning an accumulation of pus in the pleural cavity is emphyema.

    _____

7.38. The medical name for the disease commonly known as whooping cough is pertussosis.

    _____

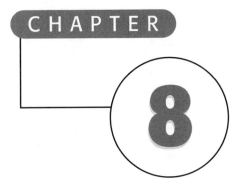

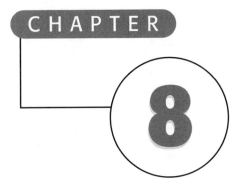CHAPTER

8

The Digestive System

LEARNING EXERCISES

Grade _____ Name _____

MATCHING WORD PARTS 1

Write the correct answer in the middle column.

Definition	Correct Answer	Possible Answers
8.1. anus	_____	enter/o
8.2. bile, gall	_____	an/o
8.3. large intestine	_____	cec/o
8.4. cecum	_____	chol/e
8.5. small intestine	_____	col/o

MATCHING WORD PARTS 2

Write the correct answer in the middle column.

Definition	Correct Answer	Possible Answers
8.6. stomach	_____	-lithiasis
8.7. liver	_____	gastr/o
8.8. gallbladder	_____	esophag/o
8.9. esophagus	_____	hepat/o
8.10. presence of stones	_____	cholecyst/o

MATCHING WORD PARTS 3

Write the correct answer in the middle column.

Definition	Correct Answer	Possible Answers
8.11. sigmoid colon	_____	-pepsia
8.12. anus and rectum	_____	pancreat/o
8.13. digestion	_____	proct/o
8.14. pancreas	_____	rect/o
8.15. rectum	_____	sigmoid/o

DEFINITIONS

Select the correct answer and write it on the line provided.

8.16. The use of a speculum to visually examine the anal canal and lower rectum is known as a/an

_____.

    anoscopy   colonoscopy   proctoscopy   sigmoidoscopy

8.17. The _____ glands are located on the face in front of each ear.

    maxillary   parotid   sublingual   submandibular

8.18. The _____ are the posterior teeth used for grinding and chewing.

    canines   cuspids   incisors   molars

8.19. The liver removes excess _____ from the bloodstream.

    bilirubin   glucose   glycogen   lipase

8.20. The gallbladder stores _____ for later use.

    bile   glycogen   hydrochloric acid   pepsin

8.21. The duodenum is part of the _____.

    cecum   large intestine   small intestine   stomach

8.22. The process of breaking down substances is known as _____.

    anabolism   catabolism   defecation   dentition

8.23. The receptors of taste are located on the _____.

    hard palate   rugae   tongue   uvula

8.24. Each tooth is surrounded by specialized mucous membrane known as the

_____.

    cementum   dentin   gingiva   pulp

8.25. The condition characterized by the telescoping of one part of the intestine into another is called

_____.

    borborygmus   flatus   intussusception   volvulus

MATCHING STRUCTURES

Write the correct answer in the middle column.

Definition	Correct Answer	Possible Answers
8.26. connects the small and large intestine	_____	cecum
8.27. major part of the large intestine leading into the rectum	_____	ileum
8.28. last division of the large intestine	_____	jejunum
8.29. middle portion of the small intestine	_____	rectum
8.30. last portion of the small intestine	_____	sigmoid colon

WHICH WORD?

Select the correct answer and write it on the line provided.

8.31. The word that means vomiting blood is _____.

hematemesis   hyperemesis

8.32. The type of hepatitis that is transmitted by contaminated food and water is _____.

hepatitis A   hepatitis B

8.33. An often fatal form of food poisoning is _____.

bulimia   botulism

8.34. The term meaning inflammation of the small intestine is _____.

colitis   enteritis

8.35. The _____ is the structure that hangs from the free edge of the soft palate.

volvulus   uvula

SPELLING COUNTS

Find the misspelled word in each sentence. Then write that word, spelled correctly, on the line provided.

8.36. An ilectomy is the surgical removal of the last portion of the small intestine. _____

8.37. The cecum is connected to the ileum by the iliocecal sphincter. _____

8.38. The term hepatarrhaphy means to suture the liver. _____

8.39. A proctoplexy is the surgical fixation of the rectum to some adjacent tissue or organ.

_____

8.40. Hepatitus is an inflammation of the liver caused by a virus or by damage from toxic substances.

_____

MATCHING CONDITIONS

Write the correct answer in the middle column.

Definition	Correct Answer	Possible Answers
8.41. a congenital defect	_____	bulimia
8.42. a soft bacterial deposit that builds up on the teeth	_____	cleft lip
8.43. an autoimmune disorder	_____	Crohn's disease
8.44. an eating disorder	_____	dental plaque
8.45. yellow tissue discoloration	_____	jaundice

TERM SELECTION

Select the correct answer and write it on the line provided.

8.46. Surgical removal of all or part of the stomach is known as a _____.

gastrectomy   gastritis   gastroenteritis   gastrotomy

8.47. Difficulty in swallowing is known as _____.

anorexia   dyspepsia   dysphagia   pyrosis

8.48. A surgical incision into the colon is known as a _____.

colectomy   colostomy   colotomy   proctectomy

8.49. Progressive degeneration of the liver is caused by the disease called _____.

cirrhosis   hepatomegaly   hepatitis   hepatorrhexis

8.50 The pigment produced by the destruction of hemoglobin in the liver is called _____.

bile   bilirubin   hydrochloric acid   pancreatic juice

SENTENCE COMPLETION

Write the correct term on the line provided.

8.51. The folds in the mucosa lining the mouth and of the stomach are known as

_____.

8.52. The return of swallowed food to the mouth is called _____.

8.53. A yellow discoloration of the skin caused by greater than normal amounts of bilirubin in the blood is called

_____.

8.54. The flow from the stomach to the duodenum is controlled by the _____

sphincter.

8.55. The medical term for the solid body wastes that are expelled through the rectum is/are

_____.

TRUE/FALSE

If the statement is true, write **T** on the line. If the statement is false, write **F** on the line.

8.56. _____ Amebic dysentery is an intestinal disease caused by Entamoeba histolytica.

8.57. _____ Hepatitis B can be prevented through immunization.

8.58. _____ Bruxism means to be without natural teeth.

8.59. _____ Gastrorrhagia means the excessive flow of gastric secretions.

8.60. _____ Eructation is the act of belching or raising gas orally from the stomach.

8.61. _____ Cholelithiasis is the presence of stones in the large intestine.

8.62. _____ Fatty substances in a stool sample indicate a parasite problem.

8.63. _____ Periodontitis is the progressive destruction of dental enamel.

8.64. _____ Pica is a craving for nonnutritional substances such as clay.

8.65. _____ A choledocholithotomy is an incision in the common bile duct for the removal of gallstones.

CLINICAL CONDITIONS

Write the correct answer on the line provided.

8.66. James Ridgeview was treated for the temporary stoppage of intestinal peristalsis. The medical term for this condition is _____.

8.67. Chang Hoon suffers from an inflammation of the stomach. The medical term for this condition is _____.

8.68. Dr. Martinson described the patient as being _____, which means he was without natural teeth.

8.69. Baby Kilgore was vomiting almost continuously. The medical term for this excessive vomiting is _____.

8.70. A/An _____ was performed on Mr. Gonzalez to create an opening between his colon and body surface.

8.71. After eating, Mr. Delahanty often suffers from heartburn. The medical term for this condition is _____.

8.72. Catherine Baldwin's presenting symptom was the passage of black stools containing digested blood. The medical term for this condition is _____.

8.73. Alberta Roberts was diagnosed as having an inflammation of one or more diverticulum. The medical term for this condition is _____.

8.74. Jason Norton suffers from _____ labialis, which is also known as cold sores.

8.75. Lisa Wilson saw her dentist because she was concerned about bad breath. Her dentist refers to this condition as _____.

WHICH IS THE CORRECT MEDICAL TERM?

Select the correct answer and write it on the line provided.

8.76. The _____ test detects hidden blood in the stools.

anoscopy   colonoscopy   enema   hemoccult

8.77. In a patient with a colostomy, the effluent flows from the _____.

colon   ileus   rectum   stoma

8.78. The term meaning the lack or loss of appetite is _____.

anorexia   bulimia   nervosa   pica

8.79. The hardened deposit on the teeth that irritates the surrounding tissues is known as

_____.

calculus   caries   gingiva   plaque

8.80. The surgical repair of the rectum is a/an _____.

anoplasty   palatoplasty   proctopexy   proctoplasty

CHALLENGE WORD BUILDING

These terms are *not* found in this chapter; however, they are made up of the following familiar word parts. You may want to look in the textbook glossary or use a medical dictionary to check your answers.

enter/o	-algia
esophag/o	-ectomy
gastr/o	-itis
hepat/o	-megaly
proct/o	-ic
sigmoid/o	-pexy
	-rrhaphy

8.81. The term meaning to suture an injured stomach is _____.

8.82. The term meaning pain in the esophagus is _____.

8.83. The term meaning the surgical removal of all or part of the sigmoid colon is

_____.

8.84. The term meaning pain in and around the anus and rectum is _____.

8.85. The term meaning the surgical fixation of the stomach to correct displacement is

_____.

8.86. The term meaning inflammation of the sigmoid colon is _____.

8.87. The term meaning the surgical removal of all or part of the esophagus and stomach is

_____.

8.88. The term referring to the liver and intestines is _____.

8.89. The term meaning abnormal enlargement of the liver is _____.

8.90. The term meaning inflammation of the stomach, small intestine, and large intestine is

_____.

LABELING EXERCISES

Identify the numbered items on the accompanying figure.

8.91. _____ glands

8.92. _____

8. 93. _____

8. 94. _____

8. 95. _____

8.96. _____

8.97. _____ intestine

8.98. vermiform _____

8.99. _____ intestine

8.100. _____ and anus

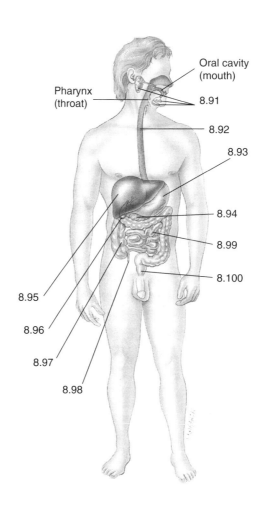

The Urinary System

LEARNING EXERCISES

Grade _____ Name _____

MATCHING WORD PARTS 1

Write the correct answer in the middle column.

Definition	Correct Answer	Possible Answers
9.1. bladder	_____	-cele
9.2. glomerulus	_____	cyst/o
9.3. hernia, tumor, cyst	_____	glomerul/o
9.4. kidney	_____	lith/o
9.5. stone, calculus	_____	nephr/o

MATCHING WORD PARTS 2

Write the correct answer in the middle column.

Definition	Correct Answer	Possible Answers
9.6. drooping down	_____	-lysis
9.7. setting free, separation	_____	-pexy
9.8. surgical fixation	_____	pyel/o
9.9. renal pelvis	_____	-ptosis
9.10. to crush	_____	-tripsy

MATCHING WORD PARTS 3

Write the correct answer in the middle column.

Definition	Correct Answer	Possible Answers
9.11. urination	_____	dia-
9.12. ureter	_____	ureter/o
9.13. urethra	_____	-ectasis
9.14. complete, through	_____	-uria
9.15. enlargement, stretching	_____	urethr/o

DEFINITIONS

Select the correct answer and write it on the line provided.

9.16. Urine is carried from the kidneys to the urinary bladder by the _____.

glomeruli   nephrons   urethras   ureters

9.17. The condition of having a stone in the urinary bladder is _____.

cholelithiasis   cystolithiasis   nephrolithiasis   ureterolithiasis

9.18. The increased excretion of urine is known as _____.

anuria   diuresis   dysuria   oliguria

9.19. Before entering the ureters, urine collects in the _____.

glomeruli   renal cortex   renal pelvis   urinary bladder

9.20. The flow of urine from the bladder is controlled by the _____.

urethral meatus   urinary meatus   urinary sphincters   urinary strictures

9.21. Urine gets its normal yellow-amber or straw color from the pigment known as

_____.

albumin   bilirubin   hemoglobin   urochrome

9.22. In the male, the _____ carries both urine and semen.

nephron   renal pelvis   ureter   urethra

9.23. A specialist who treats the genitourinary system of males is a/an _____.

gynecologist   nephrologist   neurologist   urologist

9.24. In _____, the urethral opening is on one side of the penis.

epispadias   hyperspadias   hypospadias   paraspadias

9.25. A/An _____ is a band of fibers that holds structures together abnormally.

adhesion   distention   stricture   suppuration

MATCHING STRUCTURES

Write the correct answer in the middle column.

Definition	Correct Answer	Possible Answers
9.26. the portion of a nephron active in filtering urine	_____	glomerulus
9.27. carries urine from a kidney to the urinary bladder	_____	meatus
9.28. external opening of the urethra	_____	renal cortex
9.29. outer layer of the kidney	_____	ureter
9.30. tube from the bladder to the outside of the body	_____	urethra

WHICH WORD?

Select the correct answer and write it on the line provided.

9.31. A surgical incision into the renal pelvis is _____.

   pyelotomy   pyeloplasty

9.32. The discharge of blood from the ureter is _____.

   ureterorrhagia   urethrorrhagia

9.33. The term meaning excessive urination is _____.

   incontinence   polyuria

9.34. The term meaning an inflammation of the bladder is _____.

   cystitis   pyelitis

9.35. The major waste product of protein metabolism is _____.

   urea   urine

SPELLING COUNTS

Find the misspelled word in each sentence. Then write that word, spelled correctly, on the line provided.

9.36. Urinoalysis is the examination of the physical and chemical properties of urine to determine the presence of abnormal elements. _____

9.37. Incontinance means being unable to control excretory functions. _____

9.38. Catherozation is the process used to withdraw urine from the bladder. _____

9.39. Cystorhagia is bleeding from the bladder. _____

9.40. Glomeronephritis is an inflammation of the kidney involving primarily the glomeruli.

   _____

Name _____

MATCHING ABBREVIATIONS

Write the correct answer in the middle column.

Definition	Correct Answer	Possible Answers
9.41. nephrotic syndrome	_____	ESWL
9.42. hemodialysis	_____	CRF
9.43. extracorporeal shock-wave lithotripsy	_____	HD
9.44. intravenous pyelogram	_____	NS
9.45. chronic renal failure	_____	IVP

TERM SELECTION

Select the correct answer and write it on the line provided.

9.46. The term meaning the complete stopping of urine formation by the kidneys is

_____.

anuria   nocturia   oliguria   polyuria

9.47. The term meaning suturing of the bladder is _____.

cystorrhaphy cystorrhagia cystorrhexis nephrorrhaphy

9.48. The term meaning the freeing of a kidney from adhesions is _____.

nephrolithiasis nephrolysis nephropyosis pyelitis

9.49. The term meaning scanty urination is _____.

diuresis   dysuria   enuresis   oliguria

9.50. The process of artificially filtering waste products from the patient's blood is known as

_____.

diuresis hemodialysis homeostasis hydroureter

SENTENCE COMPLETION

Write the correct term on the line provided.

9.51. An incision of the urinary meatus to enlarge the opening is a/an _____.

9.52. A stone lodged in a ureter is a/an _____.

9.53. The surgical creation of a permanent opening of the urethra is a/an _____.

9.54. The surgical fixation of the bladder to the abdominal wall is a/an _____.

9.55. Urination is also known as voiding or _____.

TRUE/FALSE

If the statement is true, write **T** on the line. If the statement is false, write **F** on the line.

9.56. _____ The ureters are about 10 to 12 inches long.

9.57. _____ The urinary bladder is located in the posterior portion of the pelvic cavity.

9.58. _____ A glomerulus consists of a cluster of capillaries.

9.59. _____ The medulla is the outer layer of the kidney.

9.60. _____ Distention means enlarged.

9.61. _____ The male urethra is approximately 1.5 inches long.

9.62. _____ Urine is formed by the processes of filtration, reabsorption, and secretion.

9.63. _____ The female urethra conveys both urine and the menstrual flow.

9.64. _____ A cystolith is a hernia of the urinary bladder.

9.65. _____ Hydronephrosis is the dilation of the pelvis and calices of one or both kidneys resulting from obstruction to the flow of urine.

CLINICAL CONDITIONS

Write the correct answer on the line provided.

9.66. Mrs. Baldridge suffers from excessive urination during the night. The medical term for this is

_____.

9.67. The surgery for Rosita LaPinta included surgical repair of the urethra. This procedure is called

_____.

9.68. Doris Volk has a chronic bladder condition involving inflammation within the wall of the bladder. This is

known as _____ cystitis.

9.69. John Danielson is being treated for abnormal narrowing of the ureter. This condition is known as

_____.

9.70. Norman Smith was born with the opening of the urethra on the upper surface of the penis. This is called

_____.

9.71. Ralph Clark's form of dialysis involves the removal of waste from his blood through a fluid exchange in the

_____ cavity.

9.72. Roberta Gridley is scheduled for surgical repair of damage to the ureter. This procedure is a/an

_____.

9.73. Letty Harding's physician ordered an IVP. The full name of this diagnostic x-ray study is an intravenous

_____.

9.74. Mr. Morita was diagnosed as having an inflammation of the kidney. The medical term for this condition is

_____.

9.75. Mrs. Franklin has a kidney stone. Rather than operate, the doctor used _____

to destroy the stone.

WHICH IS THE CORRECT MEDICAL TERM?

Select the correct answer and write it on the line provided.

9.76. The term that means a hernia of the bladder through the vaginal wall is _____.

cystocele   cystolith   cystopexy   vesicovaginal
                                                                                       fissure

9.77. The term meaning the inability to empty the bladder is _____.

incontinence   dysuria   enuresis   urinary retention

9.78. The term meaning the distention of the ureter with urine due to blockage from any cause is

_____.

homeostasis   hydroureter   ureterolith   ureterostenosis

9.79. The term meaning pain in the urethra is _____.

cystodynia   nephralgia   urethralgia   ureteralgia

9.80. A specialist in diagnosing and treating diseases and disorders of the kidneys is a/an

_____.

internist   nephrologist   proctologist   urologist

CHALLENGE WORD BUILDING

These terms are *not* found in this chapter; however, they are made up of the following familiar word parts. You may want to look in the textbook glossary or use a medical dictionary to check your answers.

cyst/o	-cele
nephr/o	-itis
pyel/o	-lysis
ureter/o	- malacia
urethr/o	- ostomy
	- otomy
	-plasty
	-ptosis
	-rrhexis
	-sclerosis

9.81. The creation of an artificial opening between the urinary bladder and the exterior of the body is a/an

_____.

9.82. A surgical incision into the kidney is a/an _____.

9.83. The term meaning abnormal hardening of the kidney is _____.

9.84. The term meaning prolapse of the bladder into the urethra is _____.

9.85. A hernia in the urethral wall is a/an _____.

9.86. The procedure to separate adhesions around a ureter is _____.

9.87. The term meaning abnormal softening of the kidney is _____.

9.88. The term meaning an inflammation of the renal pelvis and kidney is _____.

9.89. The term meaning rupture of the bladder is _____.

9.90. The term meaning surgical repair of the bladder is _____.

LABELING EXERCISES

Identify the numbered items on the accompanying figure.

9.91. _____ gland

9.92. right _____

9.93. inferior _____

9.94. renal _____

9.95. renal _____

9.96. abdominal _____

9.97. _____

9.98. urinary _____

9.99. _____

9.100. urethral _____

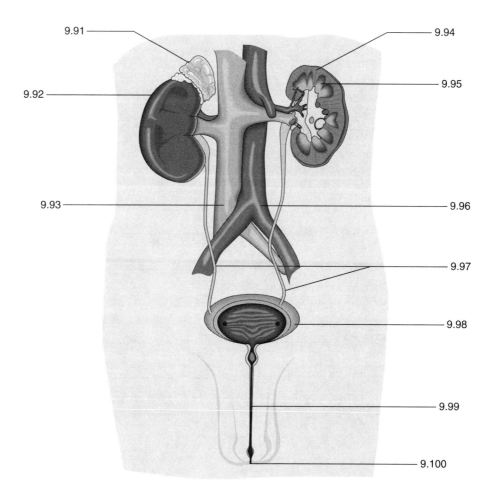

10

The Nervous System

LEARNING EXERCISES

Grade _____   Name _____

MATCHING WORD PARTS 1

Write the correct answer in the middle column.

Definition	Correct Answer	Possible Answers
10.1. brain	_____	ambul/o
10.2. bruise	_____	concuss/o
10.3. shaken together	_____	contus/o
10.4. sound	_____	ech/o
10.5. to walk	_____	encephal/o

MATCHING WORD PARTS 2

Write the correct answer in the middle column.

Definition	Correct Answer	Possible Answers
10.6. brain covering	_____	-esthesia
10.7. sensation, feeling	_____	cephal/o
10.8. spinal cord	_____	klept/o
10.9. to steal	_____	mening/o
10.10. head	_____	myel/o

MATCHING WORD PARTS 3

Write the correct answer in the middle column.

Definition	Correct Answer	Possible Answers
10.11. abnormal fear	_____	narc/o
10.12. mind	_____	neur/o
10.13. nerve	_____	-phobia
10.14. sleep	_____	psych/o
10.15. stupor	_____	somn/o

DEFINITIONS

Select the correct answer and write it on the line provided.

10.16. The term that describes the space between two neurons or between a neuron and a receptor is

_____.

    dendrite   ganglion   plexus   synapse

10.17. The protective covering over some nerve cells is the _____.

    myelin sheath   neuroglia   neurotransmitter   pia mater

10.18. The rootlike structures of a nerve that receive impulses and conduct them to the cell body are the

_____.

axons   dendrites   ganglions   terminal end fibers

10.19. The layer of the meninges that is located nearest the brain and spinal cord is the

_____.

arachnoid membrane   dura mater   meninx   pia mater

10.20. Seven vital body functions are controlled by the _____.

cerebral cortex   cerebellum   hypothalamus   thalamus

10.21. The division of the autonomic nervous system that is concerned with body functions under stress is the

_____ nervous system.

cranial   parasympathetic   peripheral   sympathetic

10.22. A network of intersecting nerves and blood or lymphatic vessels is a _____.

ganglion   plexus   synapse   tract

10.23. The cranial nerves are part of the _____ nervous system.

autonomic   central   cranial   peripheral

10.24. Motor functions are controlled by the _____ lobe of the cerebrum.

frontal   occipital   parietal   temporal

10.25. Impulses are carried away from the brain and spinal cord by the _____

neurons.

afferent   associative   connecting   efferent

MATCHING STRUCTURES

Write the correct answer in the middle column.

Definition	Correct Answer	Possible Answers
10.26. where nerves cross over	_____	cerebellum
10.27. uppermost layer of the brain	_____	cerebrum
10.28. most protected brain part	_____	hypothalamus
10.29. coordinates muscular activity	_____	medulla oblongata
10.30. controls vital body functions	_____	pons

WHICH WORD?

Select the correct answer and write it on the line provided.

10.31. A physician who specializes in administering anesthetic agents is an _____.

   anesthetist   anesthesiologist

10.32. A lowered level of consciousness marked by listlessness and drowsiness is described as

   _____.

   apathy   stupor

10.33. A disturbance in the memory marked by the inability to recall past experiences is known as

   _____.

   amnesia   aphasia

10.34. A sense perception that has no basis in external stimulation is a/an _____.

   delusion   hallucination

10.35. An excessive fear of heights is _____.

   acrophobia   agoraphobia

SPELLING COUNTS

Find the misspelled word in each sentence. Then write that word, spelled correctly, on the line provided.

10.36. A miagraine headache is characterized by sudden, severe, sharp headache that is usually present only on one side. _____

10.37. Altzheimer's disease is a group of disorders associated with degenerative changes ,including progressive memory loss, impaired thinking, and personality changes. _____

10.38. An anesthethic is the medication administered to block the normal sensation of pain.

_____

10.39. Epalepsy is a group of neurologic disorders characterized by recurrent episodes of convulsive seizure.

_____

10.40. Schiatica is a nerve inflammation that may result in pain through the thigh and leg.

_____

MATCHING ABBREVIATIONS

Write the correct answer in the middle column.

Definition	Correct Answer	Possible Answers
10.41. Parkinson's disease	_____	CP
10.42. multiple sclerosis	_____	CVA
10.43. cerebral palsy	_____	MS
10.44. tetanus	_____	PD
10.45. cerebrovascular accident	_____	tet

TERM SELECTION

Select the correct answer and write it on the line provided.

10.46. A patient with a high fever who is confused, disoriented, and unable to think clearly is suffering from

_____.

delirium   dementia   lethargy   stupor

10.47. The term meaning inflammation of the spinal cord is _____.

encephalitis   myelitis   myelosis   radiculitis

10.48. The medical term for the condition commonly known as sleepwalking is

_____.

narcolepsy   sleep apnea   somnambulism   somnolence

10.49. Trigeminal neuralgia is also known as _____.

Bell's palsy   Guillain-Barré syndrome   Lou Gehrig's disease   tic douloureux

10.50. The medical term for the condition commonly known as a reading disorder is

_____.

attention deficit disorder   autism   dyslexia   mental retardation

SENTENCE COMPLETION

Write the correct term on the line provided.

10.51. The general term used to describe bruising of brain tissue as a result of a head injury is a cerebral

_____.

10.52. A feeling of apprehension, tension, or uneasiness that stems from the anticipation of danger, the source of which is largely unknown or unrecognized, is a/an _____ state.

10.53. The term used to describe a disorder characterized by a recurrent failure to resist impulses to set fires is

_____.

10.54. _____ syndrome by proxy is a form of child abuse.

10.55. Medication that is administered to prevent or relieve depression is known as a/an

_____.

TRUE/FALSE

If the statement is true, write **T** on the line. If the statement is false, write **F** on the line.

10.56. _____ Causalgia is an intense burning pain following an injury to a sensory nerve.

10.57. _____ A cephalocele is the rupture of the membranes of the brain and spinal cord.

10.58. _____ Post-polio syndrome occurs in older patients who have had poliomyelitis.

10.59. _____ The nerves that control the left side of the body are found in the right side of the brain.

10.60. _____ Electroencephalography produces a picture of the structures of the brain.

10.61. _____ In a hemorrhagic stroke, a blood vessel in the brain leaks or ruptures.

10.62. _____ Demyelination is the destruction or loss of the myelin sheath from myelinated fibers.

10.63. _____ A sedative depresses the CNS and produces sleep.

10.64. _____ A pattern of repeated hand washing is a bipolar disorder.

10.65. _____ Tic douloureux is an inflammation of the trigeminal nerve.

CLINICAL CONDITIONS

Write the correct answer on the line provided.

10.66. Harvey Ikeman's chart listed him as being _____. This means that he is in a
coma.

10.67. After an auto accident, Anthony DeNatali required _____ to suture the ends
of a severed nerve in his hand.

10.68. George Houghton suffered a transient _____ attack (TIA). Sometimes this is a
warning of a stroke.

10.69. Ted Duncan had Parkinson's disease. To control the tremors, his doctor performed a/an
_____. This is a surgical incision into the thalamus.

10.70. Mary Beth Cawthorn was diagnosed as having _____, which is also known
as MS. This autoimmune disease is characterized by patches of demyelinated nerve fibers.

10.71. Joanne Ladner suffers from recurrent uncontrollable seizures of drowsiness and sleep. Her doctor diagnosed this condition as _____.

10.72. After her stroke, Mildred Carson was unable to understand written or spoken words. This condition is called

_____.

10.73. Jill Beck said she fainted. The medical term for this brief loss of consciousness caused by a lack of oxygen in the brain is _____.

10.74. The Baily baby was born with _____. This condition is an abnormally increased amount of cerebrospinal fluid within the brain.

10.75. After the accident, the MRI indicated that Juan Ramirez had a collection of blood trapped in the tissues of the brain. This condition is called a cranial _____.

WHICH IS THE CORRECT MEDICAL TERM?

Select the correct answer and write it on the line provided.

10.76. The term that describes an intense, burning pain after an injury to a sensory nerve is

_____.

| causalgia | hyperesthesia | hypoesthesia | paresthesia |

10.77. Medication that usually produces sleep is known as a/an _____.

| analgesic | barbiturate | hypnotic | sedative |

10.78. A/An _____ disorder is a mental condition characterized by a change in function that suggests a physical disorder but has no physical cause.

| anxiety | conversion | panic | posttraumatic stress |

10.79. Only the surface of the tissues is affected when a/an _____ anesthetic is administered.

| epidural | local | regional | topical |

10.80. To control convulsions, _____ may be administered.

| amobarbital | analgesics | phenobarbital | sedatives |

CHALLENGE WORD BUILDING

These terms are *not* found in this chapter; however, they are made up of the following familiar word parts. You may want to look in the textbook glossary or use a medical dictionary to check your answers.

poly-	encephal/o	-algia
	mening/o	-itis
	myel/o	-malacia
	neur/o	-oma
		-pathy

10.81. The term meaning pain in a nerve or nerves is _____.

10.82. The term meaning abnormal softening of the meninges is known as _____.

10.83. The term used to describe benign neoplasms made up of neurons and nerve fibers is a/an

_____.

10.84. The term meaning any degenerative disease of the brain is _____.

10.85. The term meaning an inflammation affecting many nerves is _____.

10.86. The term meaning abnormal softening of nerve tissue is known as _____.

10.87. The term meaning inflammation of the meninges and the brain is _____.

10.88. The term meaning any pathological condition of the spinal cord is _____.

10.89. The term meaning abnormal softening of the brain is _____.

10.90. The term meaning inflammation of the meninges, brain, and spinal cord is

_____.

LABELING EXERCISES

Identify the numbered items on the accompanying figures.

10.91. _____ cortex

10.92. _____ lobe

10.93. _____ lobe

10.94. _____ lobe

10.95. _____ lobe

10.96. _____

10.97. _____ callosum

10.98. _____

10.99. _____ oblongata

10.100. _____ cord

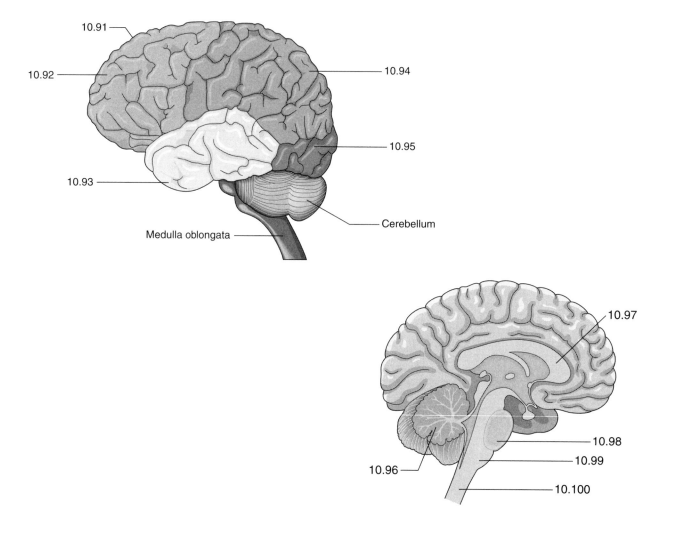

CHAPTER 11

The Special Senses: The Eyes and Ears

LEARNING EXERCISES

Grade _____ Name _____

MATCHING WORD PARTS 1

Write the correct answer in the middle column.

Definition	Correct Answer	Possible Answers
11.1. cornea, hard	_____	blephar/o
11.2. to measure	_____	-cusis
11.3. eyelid	_____	kerat/o
11.4. hearing	_____	dacryocyst/o
11.5. tear sac	_____	-metry

MATCHING WORD PARTS 2

Write the correct answer in the middle column.

Definition	Correct Answer	Possible Answers
11.6. eye, vision	_____	pseud/o
11.7. false	_____	irid/o
11.8. iris of the eye	_____	-opia
11.9. old age	_____	ophthalm/o
11.10. vision condition	_____	presby/o

MATCHING WORD PARTS 3

Write the correct answer in the middle column.

Definition	Correct Answer	Possible Answers
11.11. retina	_____	ot/o
11.12. hard, white of eye	_____	retin/o
11.13. turn	_____	scler/o
11.14. ear	_____	tympan/o
11.15. eardrum	_____	trop/o

DEFINITIONS

Select the correct answer and write it on the line provided.

11.16. The structure that maintains the shape of the eye and protects the delicate inner tissues is the

_____.

choroid   conjunctiva   cornea   sclera

Name _____

11.17. The structure that is a spiral-shaped passage leading from the oval window of the inner ear is the

_____.

cochlea   eustachian tube   organ of Corti   semicircular canal

11.18. The structure also known as the blind spot is the _____.

fovea centralis   macula lutea   optic disk   optic nerve

11.19. The structure that lies between the outer ear and the middle ear is the _____.

mastoid process   oval window   pinna   tympanic
                                                                             membrane

11.20. The structure that separates the middle ear from the inner ear is the _____.

eustachian tube   inner canthus   oval window   tympanic
                                                                             membrane

11.21. The auditory ossicle, which is also known as the anvil, is the _____.

incus   labyrinth   malleus   stapes

11.22. The term meaning lessening of the accommodation of the lens that occurs normally with aging is

_____.

ametropia   amblyopia   presbyopia   presbycusis

11.23. The term that describes reattachment of a detached retina by using a laser is

_____.

keratoplasty   laser trabeculoplasty   photorefractive keratectomy retinopexy

11.24. The term meaning turning inward of the edge of the eyelid is _____.

ectropion   emmetropia   entropion   esotropia

11.25. The condition of _____ otitis media involves a buildup of pus in the middle
       ear.

acute   effusive   purulent   serous

MATCHING CONDITIONS

Write the correct answer in the middle column.

Definition	Correct Answer	Possible Answers
11.26. squint	_____	diplopia
11.27. nearsightedness	_____	esotropia
11.28. farsightedness	_____	hyperopia
11.29. double vision	_____	myopia
11.30. cross-eyes	_____	strabismus

WHICH WORD?

Select the correct answer and write it on the line provided.

11.31. The turning outward of an eyelid is called _____.

    ectropion   entropion

11.32. The term meaning bleeding from the ears is _____.

    otorrhagia   otorrhea

11.33. The surgical placement of a ventilating tube through the eardrum to drain fluid is a

    _____.

    myringotomy   tympanostomy

11.34. A visual field test to determine losses in peripheral vision is used to diagnose

    _____.

    cataracts   glaucoma

11.35. A hearing test that involves both ears is _____.

    binaural   binocular

SPELLING COUNTS

Find the misspelled word in each sentence. Then write that word, spelled correctly, on the line provided.

11.36. The euctachian tubes lead from the middle ear to the pharynx. _____

11.37. Cerunem, which is also known as earwax, is secreted by glands that line the external auditory canal. _____

11.38. An astegmatism is a condition in which the eye does not focus properly because of unequal curvatures of the cornea. _____

11.39. The surgical procedure in which a new opening is made in the labyrinth of the inner ear is known as a fenistration. _____

11.40. A Snellan chart is used to measure visual acuity. _____

MATCHING ABBREVIATIONS

Write the correct answer in the middle column.

Definition	Correct Answer	Possible Answers
11.41. both eyes	_____	AD
11.42. left ear	_____	AS
11.43. left eye	_____	OD
11.44. right ear	_____	OS
11.45. right eye	_____	OU

TERM SELECTION

Select the correct answer and write it on the line provided.

11.46. The condition known as _____ may be treated by radial keratotomy.

astigmatism   cataracts   hyperopia   myopia

11.47. The term that describes a condition in which the pupils are unequal in size is

_____.

anisocoria   choked disk   macular degeneration   synechia

11.48. The term that describes the surgical repair of the pinna of the ear is _____.

keratoplasty   myringoplasty   otoplasty   tympanoplasty

11.49. The loss of central vision is frequently caused by _____.

glaucoma   macular degeneration   presbyopia   uveitis

11.50. The condition also known as a stye is _____.

blepharoptosis   chalazion   dacryocystitis   hordeolum

SENTENCE COMPLETION

Write the correct term on the line provided.

11.51. The ability of the lens to bend light rays to help focus them on the retina is known as

_____.

11.52. A sense of whirling, dizziness, and the loss of balance is called _____.

11.53. A specialist in measuring the accuracy of vision is a/an _____.

11.54. The medical term meaning an inflammation of the cornea is _____.

11.55.The medical term for color blindness is _____.

TRUE/FALSE

If the statement is true, write **T** on the line. If the statement is false, write **F** on the line.

11.56. _____ Dacryocystitis is associated with faulty tear drainage.

11.57. _____ A sensorineural hearing loss is also known as nerve deafness.

11.58. _____ A tarsorrhaphy is the surgical repair of the eyelids.

11.59. _____ Binaural refers to hearing in both ears.

11.60. _____ Open-angle glaucoma causes severe pain and a sudden increase in eye pressure.

11.61. _____ Rods in the retina are the receptors for color.

11.62. _____ Aqueous fluid is drained through the canal of Schlemm.

11.63. _____ Scotoma is an area of absent or depressed vision surrounded by an area of normal vision.

11.64. _____ Synechia is an adhesion of the cornea to the surrounding structures.

11.65. _____ Tympanometry is a diagnostic test to measure hearing.

CLINICAL CONDITIONS

Write the correct answer on the line provided.

11.66. Following a boxing match, Jack Lawson required _____ to repair the pinna of his injured ear.

11.67. Sheila McClelland suffers from a/an _____ hearing loss because the middle ear does not conduct sound vibrations to the inner ear normally.

11.68. Edward Cooke was treated for an inflammation of mastoid cells. The medical term for this condition is _____.

11.69. Margo Wilkins was diagnosed as having deterioration of the macula lutea of the retina. The medical term for this condition is _____ _____.

11.70. Mr. Eisner suffers from a progressive hearing loss that occurs in old age. The medical term for this condition is _____.

11.71. Juan Gutierrez has an earache caused by a buildup of fluid in the middle ear. His doctor referred to this condition as serous _____ _____.

11.72. Adrienne Jacobus says she suffers from night blindness. The medical term for this condition is _____.

11.73. Maude Colson is troubled by _____, which is a ringing sound in her ears.

11.74. Paul Ogelthorpe is color blind. This condition is listed on his chart as _____.

11.75. Mrs. Liu's hearing loss was diagnosed as being caused by ankylosis of the bones of the middle ear. The medical term for this condition is _____.

WHICH IS THE CORRECT MEDICAL TERM?

Select the correct answer and write it on the line provided.

11.76. The medical term for the condition also known as choked disk is _____.

eustachitis   papilledema   tinnitus   xerophthalmia

11.77. The term describing an adhesion that binds the iris to an adjacent structure is

_____.

blepharoptosis   convergence   scleritis   synechia

11.78. The medical term that describes the condition commonly known as double vision is

_____.

ametropia   diplopia   esotropia   hemianopia

11.79. The medical term that describes the condition commonly known as farsightedness is

_____.

amblyopia   exotropia   hyperopia   myopia

11.80. The term that describes an accumulation of earwax in the auditory canal is

_____.

conjunctivitis   impacted cerumen   otitis externa   pseudophakia

CHALLENGE WORD BUILDING

These terms are *not* found in this chapter; however, they are made up of the following familiar word parts.
You may want to look in the textbook glossary or use a medical dictionary to check your answers.

blephar/o	-algia
irid/o	-ectomy
lacrim/o	-edema
ophthalm/o	-itis
labyrinth/o	-ology
retin/o	-otomy
	-pathy

11.81. The term meaning pain felt in the iris is _____.

11.82. The term meaning inflammation of the eyelid is _____.

11.83. The term meaning an incision into the iris is a/an _____.

11.84. The term meaning any disease of the retina is _____.

11.85. The term meaning the study of the eye is _____.

11.86. The term meaning swelling of the eyelid is _____.

11.87. The term meaning a surgical incision into the lacrimal duct is a/an

_____.

11.88. The term meaning the surgical removal of the labyrinth of the inner ear is a/an

_____.

11.89. The term meaning any disease of the iris is _____.

11.90. The term meaning inflammation of the retina is _____.

LABELING EXERCISES

Identify the numbered items on the accompanying figures.

11.91. _____

11.92. _____ chamber

11.93. crystalline _____

11.94. _____

11.95. _____ centralis

11.96. _____

or _____

11.97. external _____ canal

11.98. _____ membrane

11.99. _____ tube

11.100. _____

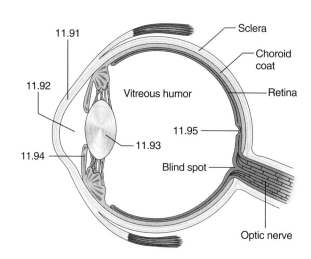

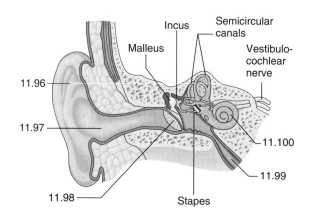

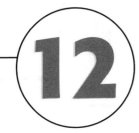

Skin: The Integumentary System

LEARNING EXERCISES

Grade _____ Name _____

MATCHING WORD PARTS 1

Write the correct answer in the middle column.

Definition	Correct Answer	Possible Answers
12.1. life	_____	albin/o
12.2. red	_____	rhytid/o
12.3. wrinkle	_____	erythr/o
12.4. sweat	_____	bi/o
12.5. white	_____	hidr/o

MATCHING WORD PARTS 2

Write the correct answer in the middle column.

Definition	Correct Answer	Possible Answers
12.6. black, dark	_____	dermat/o
12.7. fat, lipid	_____	kerat/o
12.8. lice	_____	lip/o
12.9. horny, hard	_____	melan/o
12.10. skin	_____	pedicul/o

MATCHING WORD PARTS 3

Write the correct answer in the middle column.

Definition	Correct Answer	Possible Answers
12.11. dry	_____	onych/o
12.12. fungus	_____	pil/o
12.13. hair	_____	seb/o
12.14. nail	_____	xer/o
12.15. sebum	_____	myc/o

DEFINITIONS

Select the correct answer and write it on the line provided.

12.16. The term that describes a diffuse infection of connective tissue is _____.

abscess   cellulitis   fissure   ulcer

12.17. The biopsy technique in which only part of the lesion is cut out is a/an

_____ biopsy.

excisional   exfoliative   incisional   needle

12.18. Pruritus is commonly known as _____.

    baldness   dry skin   itching   pus

12.19. An ecchymosis is commonly known as a/an _____.

    abscess   bruise   scar   ulcer

12.20. The term meaning profuse sweating is _____.

    anhidrosis   diaphoresis   hidrosis   miliaria

12.21. The term that describes a normal scar left by a wound is a _____.

    cicatrix   keloid   keratosis   papilloma

12.22. The type of treatment used to remove a port-wine stain is _____.

    abrasion   cryosurgery   laser   Mohs' chemosurgery

12.23. The removal of dirt, foreign objects, damaged tissue, and cellular debris from a wound is called

_____.

    debridement   drainage   excision   incision

12.24. A _____ degree burn has no blisters and only superficial damage to the epidermis.

    first   fourth   second   third

12.25. The lesions caused by the human papillomavirus, which are commonly known as warts, are

_____.

    nevi   petechiae   scabies   verrucae

MATCHING STRUCTURES

Write the correct answer in the middle column.

Definition	Correct Answer	Possible Answers
12.26. secrete sebum	_____	dermis
12.27. finger and toenails	_____	keratin
12.28. fibrous protein found in hair, nails, and skin	_____	mammary glands
12.29. the layer of skin below the epidermis	_____	sebaceous glands
12.30. milk-producing sebaceous glands	_____	unguis

WHICH WORD?

Select the correct answer and write it on the line provided.

12.31. The medical term for the condition commonly known as an ingrown toenail is

_____.

onychomycosis   onychocryptosis

12.32. A contagious, superficial skin infection usually seen in young children is

_____.

impetigo   xeroderma

12.33. A torn or jagged wound or an accidental cut wound is known as a _____.

laceration   lesion

12.34. Found mainly on the face, a _____ carcinoma is the most frequent but least

harmful type of skin cancer.

basal cell   squamous cell

12.35. The term meaning small pinpoint hemorrhages is _____.

petechiae   verrucae

SPELLING COUNTS

Find the misspelled word in each sentence. Then write that word, spelled correctly, on the line provided.

12.36. Soriasis is a chronic disease of the skin characterized by itching and by red papules covered with silvery scales. _____

12.37. Exema is an inflammatory skin disease with erythema, papules, and scabs.

_____

12.38. An abcess is a localized collection of pus. _____

12.39. Onyochia is an inflammation of the nail bed, resulting in the loss of the nail.

_____

12.40. Skleroderma is an autoimmune disorder that causes abnormal tissue thickening.

_____

MATCHING ABBREVIATIONS

Write the correct answer in the middle column.

Definition	Correct Answer	Possible Answers
12.41. light amplification by stimulated emission of radiation	_____	I & D
12.42. incision and draining	_____	LASER
12.43. lupus erythematosus	_____	UVA
12.44. ultraviolet B	_____	UVB
12.45. ultraviolet A	_____	LE

TERM SELECTION

Select the correct answer and write it on the line provided.

12.46. A small, knot-like swelling of granulation tissue that may result from inflammation, injury, or infection is a

_____.

cicatrix   granuloma   keratosis   petechiae

12.47. The term meaning an infestation of body lice is _____.

pediculosis capitis   pediculosis corpus   pediculosis pubis   scabies

12.48. The term meaning any redness of the skin is _____.

dermatitis   ecchymosis   erythema   urticaria

12.49. The term that describes a dry patch made up of excessive dead epidermal cells is a

_____.

bulla   macule   plaque   scale

12.50. The term that describes a cluster of boils is a _____.

acne vulgaris   carbuncle   comedo   furuncle

SENTENCE COMPLETION

Write the correct term on the line provided.

12.51. The term meaning producing or containing pus is _____.

12.52. The term meaning a fungal infection of the nail is _____.

12.53. Tissue death followed by bacterial invasion and putrefaction is known as _____.

12.54. Any condition of unusual deposits of black pigment is known as _____.

12.55. The medical term for the condition commonly known as hives is _____.

TRUE/FALSE

If the statement is true, write **T** on the line. If the statement is false, write **F** on the line.

12.56. _____ A carbon dioxide laser is used to remove tattoos.

12.57. _____ Diffuse means confined to a limited area.

12.58. _____ Dermatomycosis is a superficial fungal infection of the skin.

12.59. _____ Squamous cell carcinoma can spread quickly to other body systems.

12.60. _____ Dermatosis is any condition of the skin associated with inflammation.

12.61. _____ Putrefaction is decay that produces foul-smelling odors.

12.62. _____ A skin tag that enlarges in the elderly is malignant.

12.63. _____ The arrector pili are tiny muscles that cause the hairs to stand erect.

12.64. _____ An abnormally raised scar is known as a granuloma.

12.65. _____ A lipoma is a benign tumor made up of mature fat cells.

CLINICAL CONDITIONS

Write the correct answer on the line provided.

12.66. Robert Harris has a disease of unknown origin in which there are well-defined bald patches. Robert has a form of alopecia _____.

12.67. Jordan Caswell has an inherited deficiency or absence of pigment in the skin, hair, and eyes due to an abnormality in production of melanin. This disorder is called _____.

12.68. Mike Young hit his thumb with a hammer and soon there was a collection of blood beneath the nail. This is called a/an _____ _____.

12.69. Mrs. Higachi fell and bruised her arm. The medical term for the bruise is a/an

_____.

12.70. Rosita Chavez was diagnosed as suffering from a disorder with bleeding beneath the skin that causes spontaneous bruising. The medical term for this condition is _____.

12.71. Henry Walton was treated for a skin infection caused by the itch mite. This was entered on his chart as treatment for _____.

12.72. Dr. Liu found that Jeanette Isenberg had an abnormal skin lesion caused by excessive exposure to the sun. The medical term for this is _____ keratosis.

12.73. Mrs. Garrison had cosmetic surgery that is commonly known as a lid lift. The medical term for this treatment is a/an _____.

12.74. Tammy's teacher sent home a note alerting Tammy's parent that many of the children in the class had head lice. The medical term for this condition is _____ capitis.

12.75. Agnes Farrington uses a patch to prevent motion sickness. This is known as _____ administration.

WHICH IS THE CORRECT MEDICAL TERM?

Select the correct answer and write it on the line provided.

12.76. The term that refers to an infection of the fold of skin at the margin of a nail is

_____.

dyschromia   onychia   paronychia   vitiligo

12.77. The term for the procedure commonly known as a face lift is _____.

blepharoplasty   debridement   rhinoplasty   rhytidectomy

12.78. The form of biopsy that removes the entire lesion is a/an _____ biopsy.

cauterization   excisional   incisional   needle

12.79. The term referring to a malformation of the nail, which is also called spoon nail, is

_____.

clubbing   koilonychia   onychomycosis   paronychia

12.80. The term that describes therapy used in the treatment of spider veins is

_____.

chemical peel   dermabrasion   dermatoplasty   sclerotherapy

CHALLENGE WORD BUILDING

These terms are *not* found in this chapter; however, they are made up of the following familiar word parts. You may want to look in the textbook glossary or use a medical dictionary to check your answers.

an-	dermat/o	-derma
hypo-	hidr/o	-ectomy
	melan/o	-ia
	myc/o	-itis
	onych/o	-malacia
	py/o	-oma
	rhin/o	-osis
		-pathy
		-plasty

12.81. The term meaning abnormal softening of the nails is _____.

12.82. The term meaning an abnormal condition resulting in the diminished flow of perspiration is

_____.

12.83. The term meaning plastic surgery to change the shape or size of the nose is

_____.

12.84. The term meaning a tumor arising from the nail bed is _____.

12.85. The term meaning any pus-forming skin disease is _____.

12.86. The term meaning the surgical removal of a finger or toenail is a/an _____.

12.87. The term meaning pertaining to the absence of finger or toenails is _____.

12.88. The term meaning any disease of the skin is _____.

12.89. The term meaning any disease caused by a fungus is _____.

12.90. The term meaning that an excess of melanin is present in an area of inflammation of the skin is

_____.

LABELING EXERCISES

Identify the lesions (the numbered items) on the accompanying figures.

12.91. _____

12.92. _____

12.93. _____

12.94. _____

12.95. _____

12.96. _____

12.97. _____

12.98. _____ tissue

12.99. _____

12.100. _____ gland

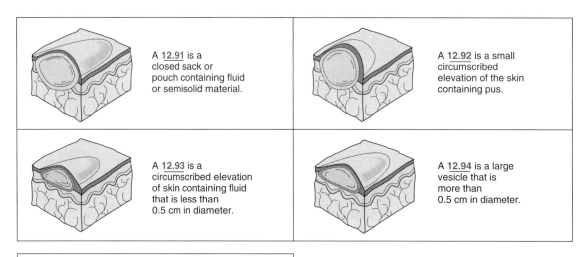

A **12.91** is a closed sack or pouch containing fluid or semisolid material.

A **12.92** is a small circumscribed elevation of the skin containing pus.

A **12.93** is a circumscribed elevation of skin containing fluid that is less than 0.5 cm in diameter.

A **12.94** is a large vesicle that is more than 0.5 cm in diameter.

A **12.95** is an open sore or erosion of the skin or mucous membrane resulting in tissue loss.

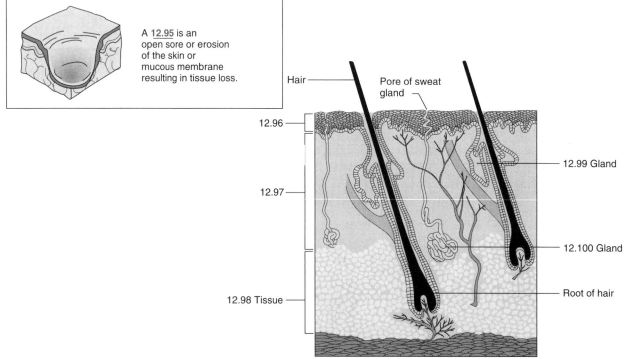

Hair

Pore of sweat gland

12.96

12.97

12.98 Tissue

12.99 Gland

12.100 Gland

Root of hair

CHAPTER 13

The Endocrine System

LEARNING EXERCISES

Grade _____ Name _____

MATCHING WORD PARTS 1

Write the correct answer in the middle column.

Definition	Correct Answer	Possible Answers
13.1. adrenal glands	_____	acr/o
13.2. extremities	_____	adren/o
13.3. ovaries or testicles	_____	crin/o
13.4. to secrete	_____	-dipsia
13.5. thirst	_____	gonad/o

MATCHING WORD PARTS 2

Write the correct answer in the middle column.

Definition	Correct Answer	Possible Answers
13.6. pituitary	_____	-ism
13.7. pineal gland	_____	pancreat/o
13.8. pancreas	_____	parathyroid/o
13.9. parathyroid	_____	pineal/o
13.10. condition	_____	pituitar/o

MATCHING WORD PARTS 3

Write the correct answer in the middle column.

Definition	Correct Answer	Possible Answers
13.11. to stimulate or act on	_____	poly-
13.12. thyroid gland	_____	somat/o
13.13. thymus, soul	_____	thym/o
13.14. many	_____	thyroid/o
13.15. body	_____	-tropin

DEFINITIONS

Select the correct answer and write it on the line provided.

13.16. The hormone that stimulates ovulation is _____.

estrogen   follicle-stimulating hormone   luteinizing hormone   progesterone

13.17. The endocrine gland known as the master gland is the _____ gland.

adrenal   hypothalamus   pituitary   thymus

13.18. The growth and secretion of the adrenal cortex is stimulated by the _____

hormone.

adrenocorticotropic   growth   melanocyte-stimulating   thyroid-stimulating

13.19. The _____ gland(s) also play(s) an important role in immune reactions.

adrenal   parathyroid   pineal   thymus

13.20. The hormone that works with the parathyroid hormone to regulate calcium levels in the blood and tissues is

_____.

aldosterone   calcitonin   glucagon   luteotropin

13.21. Cortisol is secreted by the _____.

adrenal cortex   pituitary gland   thymus   thyroid

13.22. The amount of glucose in the bloodstream is increased by the hormone

_____.

adrenaline   glucagon   hydrocortisone   insulin

13.23. Norepinephrine is secreted by the _____.

adrenal medulla   pancreatic islets   ovaries   testicles

13.24. Uterine contractions during childbirth are stimulated by the hormone _____.

estrogen   lactogenic   oxytocin   thymosin

13.25. The development of the male secondary sex characteristics is stimulated by the hormone

_____.

aldosterone   parathyroid   progesterone   testosterone

MATCHING STRUCTURES

Write the correct answer in the middle column.

Definition	Correct Answer	Possible Answers
13.26. control blood sugar levels	_____	adrenal glands
13.27. influences the sleep-wakefulness cycle	_____	pancreatic islets
13.28. regulate electrolyte levels	_____	pineal gland
13.29. stimulates metabolism	_____	pituitary gland
13.30. the master gland	_____	thyroid gland

WHICH WORD?

Select the correct answer and write it on the line provided.

13.31. Insufficient secretion of the parathyroid glands causes _____.

hyperparathyroidism   hypoparathyroidism

13.32. The growth hormone is also known as _____.

somatotropin   thyrotropin

13.33. The hormones that influence sex-related characteristics are known as _____.

glucocorticoids   gonadocorticoids

13.34. Insulin replacement therapy is always used in _____ diabetes mellitus.

type 1   type 2

13.35. An insufficient production of ADH causes _____.

diabetes insipidus   diabetes mellitus

SPELLING COUNTS

Find the misspelled word in each sentence. Then write that word, spelled correctly, on the line provided.

13.36. Metebolism is the rate at which the body uses energy and the speed at which body functions work.

_____

13.37. Diabetes melletus is a group of diseases characterized by defects in insulin production, use, or both.

_____

13.38. Hydrocortizone has an anti-inflammatory effect. _____

13.39. The hormone progestarone is released during the second half of the menstrual cycle.

_____

13.40. Thymosin is secreted by the thymas gland. _____

MATCHING ABBREVIATIONS

Write the correct answer in the middle column.

Definition	Correct Answer	Possible Answers
13.41. luteinizing hormone	_____	ACTH
13.42. glucose tolerance test	_____	GDM
13.43. lactogenic hormone	_____	GTT
13.44. adrenocorticotropic hormone	_____	LH
13.45. gestational diabetes mellitus	_____	LTH

TERM SELECTION

Select the correct answer and write it on the line provided.

13.46. A condition caused by excessive secretion of any gland is known as _____.

endocrinopathy   goiter   hypercrinism   hypocrinism

13.47. The life-threatening condition that results from the presence of excessive quantities of the thyroid hormones

is known as _____.

aldosteronism   Cushing's syndrome   Graves' disease   thyrotoxicosis

13.48. The endocrine gland located behind the sternum is the _____.

adrenal   pancreas   parathyroid   thymus

13.49. Polydipsia and polyuria are symptoms of _____.

Cushing's syndrome   diabetes insipidus   pituitary adenoma   prolactinoma

13.50. The average blood sugar over the past 3 weeks is measured by the _____ blood test.

blood sugar monitoring   fructosamine   glucose tolerance   hemoglobin A1C

SENTENCE COMPLETION

Write the correct term on the line provided.

13.51. Substances, such as sodium and potassium, that are found in the blood are known as

_____.

13.52. Calcitonin and thyroxine are secreted by the _____ gland.

13.53. Damage to the retina of the eye caused by diabetes mellitus is known as diabetic

_____.

13.54. The medical term that describes a severe form of adult hypothyroidism, with symptoms that include an enlarged tongue and puffiness of the hands and face, is _____.

13.55. Abnormal protrusion of the eyes associated with Graves' disease is known as

_____.

TRUE/FALSE

If the statement is true, write **T** on the line. If the statement is false, write **F** on the line.

13.56. _____ Pancreatalgia is an inflammation of the pancreas.

13.57. _____ Polyuria means excessive urination.

13.58. _____ Secondary aldosteronism is due to a disorder of the adrenal gland.

13.59. _____ Hypoglycemia is an abnormally decreased concentration of glucose in the blood.

13.60. _____ Gynecomastia is excessive mammary development in the male.

13.61. _____ The alpha cells of the pancreatic islets secrete insulin.

13.62. _____ Type 1 and adult-onset describe the same form of diabetes mellitus.

13.63. _____ Human chorionic gonadotropin is secreted by the adrenal cortex.

13.64. _____ The growth hormone (GH) is secreted by the pineal gland.

13.65. _____ A chemical thyroidectomy is used to treat disorders such as Graves' disease.

CLINICAL CONDITIONS

Write the correct answer on the line provided.

13.66. Grace McClelland was treated for a tumor derived from the tissue of the thymus. The medical term for this condition is a/an _____.

13.67. Joseph Butler complains of being thirsty all the time. His doctor listed this excessive thirst on his chart as _____.

13.68. During her pregnancy, Carmella DeFillipo was treated for _____ diabetes.

13.69. Linda Thomas has a progressive disease that occurs when adrenal glands do not produce enough cortisol. This condition is known as _____ disease.

13.70. Patty Edward requires daily insulin injections to control her _____ -dependent (type 1) diabetes mellitus.

13.71. When "the champ" was training for the Olympics, he was tempted to use _____ steroids to increase his strength and muscle mass.

13.72. Leigh Franklin developed a condition that is characterized by extremely large hands and feet. The medical term for this condition is _____.

13.73. As a result of a congenital lack of thyroid secretion, the Vaugh-Eames child suffers from arrested physical and mental development. The medical term for this condition is _____.

13.74. Raymond Grovenor is excessively tall and large. This condition, which was caused by excessive functioning of the pituitary gland before puberty, is known as _____.

13.75. Rose Liu required the surgical removal of her pancreas. The medical term for this procedure is a/an _____.

WHICH IS THE CORRECT MEDICAL TERM?

Select the correct answer and write it on the line provided.

13.76. Conn's syndrome is also known as _____.

hypercortisolism   hypothyroidism   primary aldosteronism   secondary aldosteronism

13.77. A benign tumor of the pituitary gland that causes the excess secretion of ACTH is known as a/an

_____.

hyperpituitarism   hypopituitarism   pituitary adenoma   prolactinoma

13.78. The autoimmune disorder that is characterized by exophthalmos is known as

_____.

Graves' disease   hypothyroidism   Hashimoto's thyroiditis   thyrotoxicosis

13.79. The condition that may progress to diabetic ketoacidosis is _____.

diabetic neuropathy   diabetic retinopathy   hyperglycemia   hypoglycemia

13.80. The hormone that plays an important role in the immune system is _____.

glucagon   melatonin   parathyroid   thymosin

CHALLENGE WORD BUILDING

These terms are *not* found in this chapter; however, they are made up of the following familiar word parts. You may want to look in the textbook glossary or use a medical dictionary to check your answers.

endo-	adren/o	-emia
	crin/o	-itis
	insulin/o	-megaly
	pancreat/o	-ology
	pineal/o	-oma
	thyroid/o	-otomy
	thym/o	-pathy

13.81. The term meaning a surgical incision into the thyroid gland is a/an _____.

13.82. The study of the endocrine glands and their secretions is known as _____.

13.83. The term meaning enlargement of the adrenal glands is _____.

13.84. The term meaning any disease of the thymus gland is _____.

13.85. The term meaning an inflammation of the thyroid gland is _____.

13.86. The term meaning a surgical incision into the pancreas is a/an _____.

13.87. The term meaning any disease of the adrenal glands is _____.

13.88. The term meaning a tumor of the pineal gland is a/an _____.

13.89. The term meaning abnormally high levels of insulin in the blood is _____.

13.90. The term meaning an inflammation of the adrenal glands is _____.

LABELING EXERCISES

Identify the numbered items on the accompanying figure.

13.91. _____ gland

13.92. _____ glands

13.93. _____ gland

13.94. _____ of the
female

13.95. _____

13.96. _____ gland

13.97. _____ gland

13.98. _____ glands

13.99. _____ islets

13.100. _____ of the
male

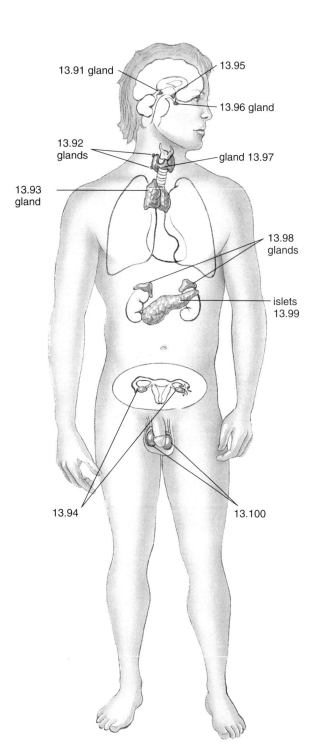

13.91 gland   13.95

13.96 gland

13.92
glands   gland 13.97

13.93
gland

13.98
glands

islets
13.99

13.94   13.100

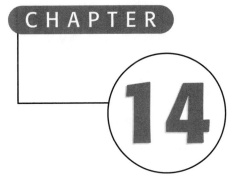

CHAPTER 14

The Reproductive Systems

LEARNING EXERCISES

Grade _____ Name _____

MATCHING WORD PARTS 1

Write the correct answer in the middle column.

Definition	Correct Answer	Possible Answers
14.1. menstruation	_____	cervic/o
14.2. pregnant	_____	colp/o
14.3. female	_____	gynec/o
14.4. vagina	_____	men/o
14.5. cervix	_____	-gravida

MATCHING WORD PARTS 2

Write the correct answer in the middle column.

Definition	Correct Answer	Possible Answers
14.6. egg	_____	metr/o
14.7. ovary	_____	ov/o
14.8. prostate	_____	oophor/o
14.9. testicle	_____	orchid/o
14.10. uterus	_____	prostat/o

MATCHING WORD PARTS 3

Write the correct answer in the middle column.

Definition	Correct Answer	Possible Answers
14.11. vulva	_____	nulli-
14.12. surgical fixation	_____	mamm/o
14.13. tube	_____	salping/o
14.14. breast	_____	-pexy
14.15. none	_____	episi/o

Name _____

DEFINITIONS

Select the correct answer and write it on the line provided.

14.16. The term that describes the inner layer of the uterus is _____.

   corpus   endometrium   myometrium   perimetrium

14.17. The term that is used to describe the fertilized egg immediately after conception is

   _____.

   embryo   fetus   gamete   zygote

14.18. Mucus to lubricate the vagina is produced by _____ glands.

   Bartholin's   bulbourethral   Cowper's   follicle

14.19. The finger-like structures of the fallopian tube that catch the ovum are the

   _____.

   fimbriae   fundus   infundibulum   oviducts

14.20. Approximately between days 15 and 28, the _____ phase of the menstrual

   cycle occurs.

   menstrual   ovulatory   postmenstrual   premenstrual

14.21. The term used to describe the normal position of the uterus is _____.

   anteflexion   anteversion   retroflexion   retroversion

14.22. The beginning of the menstrual function that begins at puberty is called _____.

   menarche   menopause   menses   menstruation

14.23. The _____ runs down the length of the testicle and then turns upward into

   the body, where it becomes a narrower tube called the vas deferens.

   ejaculatory duct   epididymis   seminal vesicle   urethra

14.24. The region between the vaginal orifice and the anus is known as the _____.

   clitoris   mons pubis   perineum   vulva

14.25. The release of a mature egg by the ovary is known as _____.

   coitus   fertilization   implantation   ovulation

MATCHING STRUCTURES

Write the correct answer in the middle column.

Definition	Correct Answer	Possible Answers
14.26. carry milk from the mammary	_____	clitoris glands
14.27. encloses the testicles	_____	lactiferous ducts
14.28. external female genitalia	_____	prepuce
14.29. protects the tip of the penis	_____	scrotum
14.30. sensitive tissue near vaginal opening	_____	vulva

WHICH WORD?

Select the correct answer and write it on the line provided.

14.31. The term used to describe a woman during her first pregnancy is a _____.

      primigravida   primipara

14.32. The fluid secreted by the breasts during the first days after giving birth is _____.

      colostrum   meconium

14.33. The term meaning inflammation of the vulva is _____.

      vulvodynia   vulvitis

14.34. The total absence of sperm in the semen is known as _____.

      azoospermia   oligospermia

14.35. A woman who has never borne a viable child is a _____.

      nulligravida   nullipara

SPELLING COUNTS

Find the misspelled word in each sentence. Then write that word, spelled correctly, on the line provided.

14.36. The prostrate gland secretes a thick fluid that aids the motility of the sperm.

_____

14.37. The normal periodic discharge from the uterus is known as menstration.

_____

14.38. The plasenta is also known as the afterbirth. _____

14.39. A Papanicola test is an exfoliative biopsy for the detection and diagnosis of conditions of the cervix and surrounding tissues. _____

14.40. The surgical removal of the foreskin of the penis is known as cercumsion.

_____

MATCHING SEXUALLY TRANSMITTED DISEASES

Write the correct answer in the middle column.

Definition	Correct Answer	Possible Answers
14.41. characterized by painful urination and an abnormal discharge	_____	genital herpes
14.42. caused by the spirochete *Treponema pallidum*	_____	gonorrhea
14.43. antiviral drugs ease symptoms but do not cure	_____	genital warts
14.44. human papilloma virus	_____	syphilis
14.45. a vaginal inflammation caused by a protozoan parasite	_____	trichomonas

TERM SELECTION

Select the correct answer and write it on the line provided.

14.46. An accumulation of pus in the fallopian tube is known as _____.

    leiomyoma   pelvic inflammatory disease   pyosalpinx   salpingitis

14.47. A varicose vein of the testicles is known as _____.

    cryptorchidism   hydrocele   phimosis   varicocele

14.48. Abnormal tipping, with the body of the uterus bent and forming an angle with the cervix, is known as

    _____.

    anteflexion   anteversion   retroflexion   retroversion

14.49. A markedly reduced menstrual flow and abnormally infrequent menstruation is called

    _____.

    amenorrhea   hypomenorrhea   oligomenorrhea   polymenorrhea

14.50. The diagnostic test that is usually performed between the eighth and tenth week of pregnancy is

    _____.

    amniocentesis   chorionic villus sampling   electronic fetal monitoring   pelvimetry

SENTENCE COMPLETION

Write the correct term on the line provided.

14.51. The dark area surrounding the nipple is known as the _____.

14.52. During delivery, when the buttocks or feet are presented first, this is known as a/an

    _____ birth.

14.53. The most serious form of toxemia of pregnancy is known as _____.

14.54. The term meaning suturing the vagina is _____.

14.55. The structure that connects the fetus to the placenta is known as the _____ cord.

TRUE/FALSE

If the statement is true, write **T** on the line. If the statement is false, write **F** on the line.

14.56. _____ When the mother's blood is Rh-negative (Rh⁻), and the father's is Rh-positive (RH⁺), the baby may inherit the Rh factor from the father.

14.57. _____ Meconium is the vaginal discharge that occurs during the first week or two after childbirth.

14.58. _____ A hysteroscope is an endoscope used for direct visual examination of the interior of the uterus.

14.59. _____ The chorion is also known as the bag of waters.

14.60. _____ Dilation is the expansion of an opening.

14.61. _____ Mittelschmerz means pain between menstrual periods and usually occurs at the time of ovulation.

14.62. _____ A PSA test is used to determine the number of sperm in a semen specimen.

14.63. _____ An Apgar score is an evaluation of a newborn infant's physical status.

14.64. _____ Hysterosalpingography is the use of ultrasound to image the uterus and fallopian tubes.

14.65. _____ An ectopic pregnancy may occur in a fallopian tube.

CLINICAL CONDITIONS

Write the correct answer on the line provided.

14.66. Mr. Romer was treated for prostatomegaly. This condition is also known as benign

_____ _____.

14.67. Mary Smith required the delivery of her baby through an incision in the maternal abdominal and uterine wall. The full medical term for this procedure is a/an _____ section.

14.68. Daniel Grossman was treated for a urethral discharge coming from the prostate gland. The medical term for this condition is _____.

14.69. Rita Cheri, who is 25, is concerned because her menstrual periods have stopped and she knows that she is not pregnant. Her doctor described this condition as _____.

14.70. To prevent laceration of the tissues during the delivery of Barbara Klein's baby, her doctor performed a/an

_____.

14.71. Early in her pregnancy, Maria Jimenez suffered a miscarriage. The medical term for this condition is a spontaneous _____.

14.72. Harriet Ingram was diagnosed as having a leiomyoma, which is a benign tumor derived from the smooth muscle of the uterus. This condition is also known as a/an _____.

14.73. Harry Belcher's doctor removed a portion of both vas deferens. The medical term for this sterilization procedure is a/an _____.

14.74. There were complications in Jane Marsall's pregnancy caused by the abnormal implantation of the placenta in the lower portion of the uterus. The medical term for this condition is placenta _____.

14.75. Immediately after birth, the Reicher baby was described as being a newborn or a/an _____.

WHICH IS THE CORRECT MEDICAL TERM?

Select the correct answer and write it on the line provided.

14.76. The fluid secreted by the breasts during the first days after giving birth is known as _____.

colostrum   involution   lochia   meconium

14.77. Excessive uterine bleeding that occurs during both the menses and at irregular intervals is known as _____.

menorrhagia   menometrorrhagia   mittelschmerz   polymenorrhea

14.78. The term that describes an inflammation of the glans penis is _____.

anorchism   balanitis   epididymitis   orchitis

14.79. The term that describes precancerous lesions of the cervix is _____.

cervical dysplasia   cervicitis   colporrhexis   vaginitis

14.80. Which term means a profuse white mucus discharge from the uterus and vagina?

endocervicitis   leukorrhea   pruritus vulvae   vaginitis

CHALLENGE WORD BUILDING

These terms are *not* found in this chapter; however, they are made up of the following familiar word parts. You may want to look in the textbook glossary or use a medical dictionary to check your answers.

endo-	hyster/o	-cele
	mast/o	-dynia
	metr/i-	itis
	oophor/o	-plasty
	vagin/o	-pexy
	vulv/o	-rrhaphy
		-rrhexis

14.81. The term meaning a hernia protruding into the vagina is _____.

14.82. The term meaning pain in the breast is _____.

14.83. The term meaning an inflammation of the endometrium is _____.

14.84. The term meaning the surgical repair of an ovary is a/an _____.

14.85. The term meaning pain in the vagina is _____.

11.86. The term meaning to suture the uterus is _____.

14.87. The term meaning a hernia of the uterus, particularly during pregnancy, is a/an

_____.

14.88. The term meaning the surgical fixation of a displaced ovary is _____.

14.89. The term meaning the rupture of the uterus, particularly during pregnancy, is

_____.

14.90. The term meaning an inflammation of the vulva and the vagina is _____.

LABELING EXERCISES

Identify the numbered items on the accompanying figures.

14.91. _____ bladder

14.92. _____ gland

14.93. _____

14.94. _____

14.95. _____

14.96. _____ tube

14.97. _____

14.98. _____ bladder

14.99. _____

14.100. _____

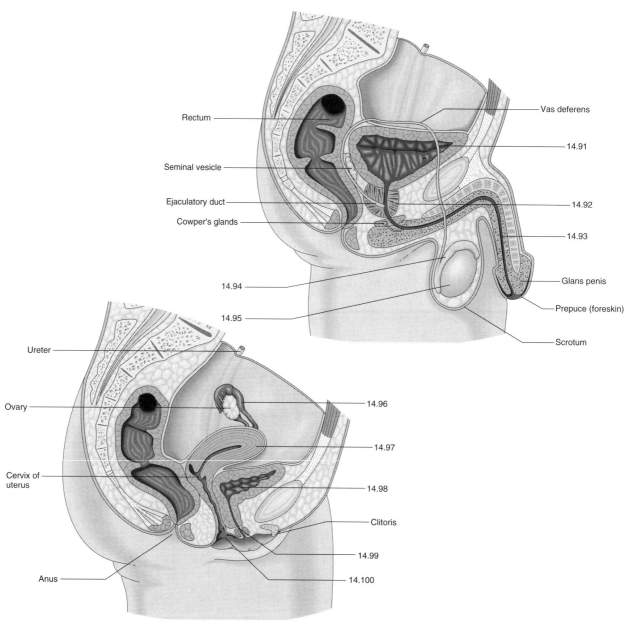

CHAPTER

15

Diagnostic Procedures and Pharmacology

LEARNING EXERCISES

Grade _____ Name _____

MATCHING WORD PARTS 1

Write the correct answer in the middle column.

Definition	Correct Answer	Possible Answers
15.1. relationship to motion	_____	albumin/o
15.2. glowing	_____	calc/i
15.3. sugar	_____	cin/e
15.4. albumin, protein	_____	fluor/o
15.5. calcium	_____	glycos/o

MATCHING WORD PARTS 2

Write the correct answer in the middle column.

Definition	Correct Answer	Possible Answers
15.6. blood	_____	-graph
15.7. pertaining to	_____	-graphy
15.8. process of recording	_____	hemat/o
15.9. resulting record or picture	_____	-ous
15.10. through	_____	per-

MATCHING WORD PARTS 3

Write the correct answer in the middle column.

Definition	Correct Answer	Possible Answers
15.11. visual examination instrument	_____	phleb/o
15.12. urine	_____	radi/o
15.13. vein	_____	-scope
15.14. visual examination	_____	-scopy
15.15. radiation	_____	-uria

DEFINITIONS

Select the correct answer and write it on the line provided.

15.16. The _____ projection has the patient positioned at right angles to the film.

anteroposterior   lateral   oblique   posteroanterior

15.17. The instrument used to examine the interior of the eye is a/an _____.

ophthalmoscope   otoscope   speculum   sphygmomano-
meter

15.18. The imaging technique that produces multiple cross-sectional images using x-radiation is

_____.

conventional x-ray   computed tomography   magnetic resonance imaging   ultrasound

15.19. The blood test used to indicate the presence of inflammation in the body is commonly known as a/an

_____ test.

agglutination   lipid   sed rate   serum enzyme

15.20. The diagnostic technique that uses the echoes of sound waves to image deep structures of the body is

_____.

cineradiography   fluoroscopy   magnetic resonance   ultrasound
                                                      imaging

15.21. The term _____ describes the presence of calcium in the urine.

albuminuria   calciuria   creatinuria   glycosuria

15.22. The _____ _____ test is used to monitor

anticoagulant therapy.

lipid panel   prothrombin time   sedimentation rate   serum enzyme

15.23. The _____ test measures the percentage by volume of packed red blood cells in a

whole blood sample.

hematocrit   hemoglobin   red blood cell count   white blood cell
                                                                                   count

15.24. An abnormal, "rattley" respiratory sound heard while listening to the chest while the patient is breathing in is

known as a _____.

bruit   rale   rhonchus   stridor

15.25. The substances formed when the body breaks down fat is/are _____.

albumin   creatinine   ketones   urea

MATCHING TECHNIQUES

Write the correct answer in the middle column.

Definition	Correct Answer	Possible Answers
15.26. uses powerful magnets	_____	centesis
15.27. uses a glowing screen	_____	CT
15.28. provides cross-sectional views	_____	x-rays
15.29. removal of fluid for diagnostic purposes	_____	fluoroscopy
15.30. shows hard tissues as white	_____	MRI

WHICH WORD?

Select the correct answer and write it on the line provided.

15.31. The term meaning an unexpected reaction to a drug is _____.

idiosyncratic   palliative

15.32. The technology that combines tomography with radionuclide traces is called

_____.

PET   radioimmunoassay

15.33. A substance that does not allow x-rays to pass through is said to be _____.

radiolucent   radiopaque

15.34. A periapical film is an example of an _____ dental radiograph.

extraoral   intraoral

15.35. The name of a _____ drug is always spelled with a capital letter.

brand name   generic

SPELLING COUNTS

Find the misspelled word in each sentence. Then write that word, spelled correctly, on the line provided.

15.36. Listening through a stethoscope for sounds within the body to determine the condition of the lungs, pleura, heart, and abdomen is known as asultation. _____

15.37. A sphygnomanometer is used to measure blood pressure. _____

15.38. The technique used to visualize body parts in motion is known as fluroscopy.

_____

15.39. The clumping together of cells or particles when mixed with incompatible blood is called agelutination.

_____

15.40. A stethescope is used to listen for sounds within the body. _____

MATCHING ABBREVIATIONS

Write the correct answer in the middle column.

Definition	Correct Answer	Possible Answers
15.41. as needed	_____	b.i.d.
15.42. four times a day	_____	NPO
15.43. nothing by mouth	_____	p.r.n.
15.44. three times a day	_____	q.i.d.
15.45. twice a day	_____	t.i.d.

TERM SELECTION

Select the correct answer and write it on the line provided.

15.46. The term meaning drawing of fluid from the sac surrounding the heart is _____.

    abdominocentesis   cardiocentesis   pericardiocentesis   thoracentesis

15.47. The term meaning the abnormal presence of blood in the urine is _____.

    albuminuria   creatinuria   hematuria   ketonuria

15.48. The term meaning a projection in which the patient is facing the film and parallel to it is

_____.

anteroposterior   lateral   oblique   posteroanterior

15.49. The term _____ describes a laboratory technique in which a radioactively labeled

substance is mixed with a blood specimen.

nuclear scan   perfusion   radioactive tracer   radioimmunoassay

15.50. The term meaning the administration of a medication by injection is _____.

parenteral   percutaneous   transcutaneous   transdermal

SENTENCE COMPLETION

Write the correct term on the line provided.

15.51. The path that the x-ray beam follows through the body from entrance to exit is known as the

_____.

15.52. When a factor in the patient's condition makes the use of a drug dangerous or ill-advised, this is known as a/an

_____.

15.53. A "murmury" sound heard in auscultation, especially an abnormal one, is known as a/an

_____.

15.54. The instrument used to visually examine the external ear and the eardrum is a/an

_____.

15.55. A compulsive, uncontrollable dependence on a substance or drug is known as a/an

_____.

TRUE/FALSE

If the statement is true, write **T** on the line. If the statement is false, write **F** on the line.

15.56. _____ Excessive exposure to x-radiation is dangerous and may cause death.

15.57. _____ A barium enema makes the stomach visible in a GI series.

15.58. _____ Compliance means that the patient has accurately followed instructions.

15.59. _____ A contrast medium makes it possible to image internal structures that otherwise cannot be seen on x-ray films.

15.60. _____ Ultrasound is used to produce images of cross-sections of the body.

15.61. _____ For an oblique projection, the patient is positioned so that his body is parallel to the film.

15.62. _____ Prothrombin time is the number of seconds required for thromboplastin to coagulate plasma.

15.63. _____ A placebo has the potential to cure a disease.

15.64. _____ An MRI can safely be recommended for a patient with a pacemaker.

15.65. _____ Nuclear medicine is used to construct a three-dimensional image of the body.

CLINICAL CONDITIONS

Write the correct answer on the line provided.

15.66. The urinalysis for Selma LaPinta showed the presence of pus. The medical term for this condition is

_____.

15.67. For the rectal examination, Mr. Johnson was placed in the _____-

_____ position, with his face down, his hips flexed, and his knees and chest resting on the table.

15.68. In preparation for Kelly Harrison's thyroid scan, radioactive _____ was administered.

15.69. During her examination of the patient, Dr. Wong used _____ to feel the texture, size, consistency, and location of certain body parts.

15.70. Dr. McDowell ordered a blood _____ _____ (BUN) test for his patient because this test is a rough indicator of kidney function.

15.71. In preparation for his upper GI series, Dwight Oshone swallowed a liquid containing the contrast medium

_____.

15.72. Maria Martinez underwent _____ to reexpand her collapsed lung.

15.73. For the examination, Scott Cunningham was placed lying on his belly with his face down. This is a/an

_____ position.

15.74. The urinalysis for Kathleen McCaffee showed the presence of glucose in the urine. The medical term for this condition is _____.

15.75. During the examination, Dr. Roberts used _____. This involves tapping the surface of the body with a finger or instrument.

WHICH IS THE CORRECT MEDICAL TERM?

Select the correct answer and write it on the line provided.

15.76. The term meaning an undesirable drug response is a/an _____ response.

adverse drug   idiosyncratic   potentiation   synergism

15.77. The examination position that is also used for the treatment of shock is the _____ position.

lithotomy   recumbent   Sims'   Trendelenburg

15.78. The type of dental radiograph that shows the entire tooth and some of the surrounding tissue is a/an _____ film.

bite-wing   extraoral   periapical   survey

15.79. The imaging technique that uses one to three gamma cameras to capture images is _____.

MRI   PET   radioimmunoassay   SPECT

15.80. The examination position that has the patient in a supine position with the feet and legs supported in stirrups is the _____ position.

decubitus   dorsal recumbent   lithotomy   Sims'

CHALLENGE WORD BUILDING

These terms are not found in this chapter; however, they are made up of the following familiar word parts. You may want to look in the textbook glossary or use a medical dictionary to check your answers.

hyper-	albumin/o	-centesis
hypo-	arthr/o	-emia
	calc/i	-gram
	cyst/o	-ology
	glycos/o	-scope
	protein/o	-scopy
	py/o	-uria
	radi/o	

15.81. The term meaning the visual examination of the interior of a joint is _____.

15.82. The term meaning an abnormally high level of albumin in the blood is _____.

15.83. The term meaning the presence of excess sugar in the urine is _____.

15.84. The instrument used to visually examine the interior of the urinary bladder is a/an

_____.

15.85. The term meaning the study of the use of radiant energy and radioactive substances in medicine is

_____.

15.86. The term meaning a surgical puncture to remove fluid from the interior of a joint is

_____.

15.87. The term meaning an abnormally low level of calcium in the circulating blood is

_____.

15.88. The term meaning the record produced by a radiographic study of blood vessels is a/an

_____.

15.89. The term meaning the presence of pus-forming organisms in the blood is _____.

15.90. The term meaning the presence of excess protein in the urine is _____.

LABELING EXERCISES

Identify the numbered items on the accompanying figures.

15.91. This is the _____
    position.

15.92. This is the _____
    recumbent position.

15.93. This is the _____
    position.

15.94. This is the _____
    recumbent position.

15.95. This is the _____
    position.

15.96. This is the _____
    position.

15.97. This is a/an _____
    injection.

15.98. This is a/an _____
    injection.

15.99. This is a/an _____
    injection.

15.100. This is a/an _____
    injection.

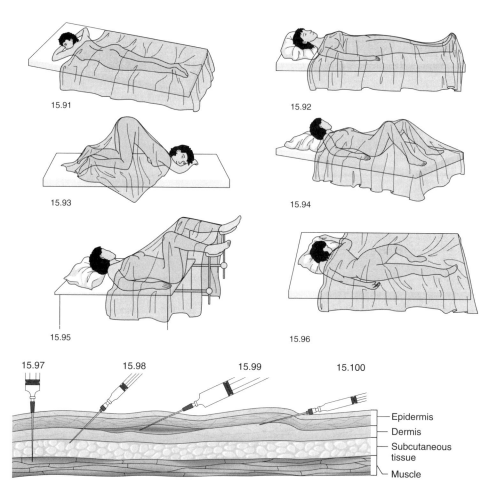

15.91

15.92

15.93

15.94

15.95

15.96

15.97   15.98   15.99   15.100

Epidermis

Dermis

Subcutaneous
tissue

Muscle

Comprehensive Medical Terminology Review

This section is designed to help you prepare for your medical terminology final examination. It contains three major parts.

- The **Study Tips** are designed to help you use your review time effectively.
- The **Review Session** contains 100 practice questions. You can review these questions as often as you want until you have mastered them.
- The **Confirming Mastery** section simulates a final test and contains 100 questions.
- **Caution**: None of the review or mastery questions are taken from the actual final test.

STUDY TIPS

USE YOUR VOCABULARY LISTS

- After you have added any terms suggested by your instructor, photocopy the vocabulary list for each chapter in your textbook. These sheets are easy to carry with you for additional review whenever you have a free minute.
- Review the terms on each list. When you have mastered a term, put a check in the box next to it. If you cannot spell and define a term, highlight it for further study.
- Look up the meanings of the highlighted terms in the textbook and work on mastering them.

USE YOUR FLASH CARDS

- Use the flash cards from the back of this workbook.
- As you go through them, remove from the stack all those word parts you can define.
- Keep working until you have mastered all of these word parts.

REVIEW YOUR LEARNING EXERCISES

You should have been saving your corrected Learning Exercise pages. Take a few minutes to go through these sheets and note where you made mistakes. Ask yourself, "*Do I know the correct answer now?*" If not, add that term or word part to your study list.

APPENDIX C

- Appendix C in your textbook contains all of the pathology and procedure terms from the textbook, plus the challenge word-building terms you encountered at the end of each chapter.
- Review the terms in these sections. Put a check mark next to the terms you know. Highlight terms you have not mastered and, next time through, concentrate on these terms.

MAKE YOUR OWN STUDY LIST

- By now you should have greatly reduced the number of terms still to be mastered. Make a list of these terms and word parts and concentrate on them.

HELP SOMEONE ELSE

- One of the greatest ways to really learn something is by teaching it! If a classmate is having trouble, tutoring that person will help both of you learn the material.

COMPREHENSIVE MEDICAL TERMINOLOGY REVIEW SESSION

Grade _____ Name _____

MATCHING WORD PARTS 1

Write the *letter* of the correct answer on the line provided.

RS.1. _____ *brady-*   **A.** abnormal condition

RS.2. _____ *colp/o*   **B.** rapid

RS.3. _____ *metr/o*   **C.** slow

RS.4. _____ *-osis*   **D.** uterus

RS.5. _____ *tachy-*   **E.** vagina

MATCHING WORD PARTS 2

Write the *letter* of the correct answer on the line provided.

RS.6. _____ *-desis*   **A.** prolapse

RS.7. _____ *-ic*   **B.** setting free

RS.8. _____ *-lysis*   **C.** surgical fixation

RS.9. _____ *-pexy*   **D.** to bind together

RS.10. _____ *-ptosis*   **E.** pertaining to

MATCHING WORD PARTS 3

Write the *letter* of the correct answer on the line provided.

RS.11. _____ *-emia*   **A.** breathing

RS.12. _____ *encephal/o*   **B.** urine

RS.13. _____ *mening/o*   **C.** blood condition

RS.14. _____ *-pnea*   **D.** brain

RS.15. _____ *-uria*   **E.** brain covering

DEFINITIONS

Circle the *letter* of the correct answer.

RS.16.   Which t-erm means the surgical removal of a joint?

   a. angiectomy

   b. arteriectomy

   c. atherectomy

   d. arthrectomy

RS.17.   Which term means the abnormal development or growth of cells?

   a. dyscrasia

   b. dyslexia

   c. dysmenorrhea

   d. dysplasia

RS.18.   Which form of anemia is a genetic disorder?

   a. aplastic anemia

   b. hemolytic anemia

   c. megaloblastic anemia

   d. sickle cell anemia

RS.19.   Which condition is characterized by rapidly worsening muscle weakness that may lead to temporary paralysis?

   a. Becker's muscular dystrophy

   b. Bell's palsy

   c. Guillain-Barré syndrome

   d. Raynaud's phenomenon

RS.20.   Which term describes a benign tumor made up of newly formed blood vessels?

   a. hemangioma

   b. hematemesis

   c. hematoma

   d. hematuria

RS.21.   Which term means slight paralysis of one side of the body?

   a. hemiparesis

   b. hemiplegia

   c. myoparesis

   d. quadriplegia

RS.22.   Which term means the surgical removal of part of the stomach and upper portion of the small intestine?

   a. esophagogastrectomy

   b. esophagoplasty

   c. gastroduodenostomy

   d. gastrostomy

RS.23. Which term describes an added sound with a musical pitch during breathing that is also known as wheezing?

a. bruit

b. rale

c. rhonchus

d. stridor

RS.24. Which term means bleeding from the bladder?

a. cystoptosis

b. cystorrhagia

c. cystorrhaphy

d. cystorrhexis

RS.25. Which skin condition is caused by a staphylococcal infection and is commonly known as a boil?

a. abscess

b. carbuncle

c. furuncle

d. pustule

MATCHING GENETIC DISORDERS

Write the *letter* of the correct answer on the line provided.

RS.26. _____ cystic fibrosis

A. Missing an essential digestive enzyme.

RS.27. _____ hemochromatosis

B. Characterized by short-lived red blood cells.

RS.28. _____ phenylketonuria

C. Causes abnormal hemoglobin.

RS.29. _____ sickle cell anemia

D. Also known as iron overload disease.

RS.30. _____ thalassemia

E. Affects the lungs and digestive system

WHICH WORD?

Circle the *correct term*.

RS.31. The term meaning the absence of normal sensitivity to pain is *anesthesia / anesthetic*.

RS.32. The term meaning any fungus infection of the nail is *onychocryptosis / onychomycosis*.

RS.33. The term meaning the ongoing presence of a disease within a population, group, or area is *endemic / pandemic*.

RS.34. The surgical stiffening of a joint or joining of spinal vertebrae is called *arthrodesis / arthrolysis*.

RS.35. The term meaning an accumulation of pus in the pleural cavity is *atelectasis / empyema*.

SPELLING COUNTS

Find the misspelled word in each sentence. Then write that *word*, spelled correctly, on the line provided.

RS.36. _____ An opthalmologist specializes in diagnosing and treating diseases and disorders of the eye.

RS.37. _____ The progressive loss of lung function due to a decrease in the total number of alveoli is known as empysema.

RS.38. _____ Altzheimer's disease is a group of disorders associated with degenerative changes in the brain structure.

RS.39. _____ The term blepharodema means swelling of the eyelid.

RS.40. _____ The term oligospermism is also known as a low sperm count.

MATCHING BONE CONDITIONS

Write the *letter* of the correct answer on the line provided.

RS.41. _____ osteomalacia   **A.** Abnormal hardening of bone.

RS.42. _____ osteonecrosis   **B.** Abnormal softening of bone.

RS.43. _____ osteoporosis   **C.** Death of bone tissue.

RS.44. _____ osteosarcoma   **D.** Loss of bone density.

RS.45. _____ osteosclerosis   **E.** Malignant bone tumor.

TERM SELECTION

Circle the *letter* of the correct answer.

RS.46. Which condition is commonly known as a bruise?
   a. ecchymosis
   b. embolus
   c. emesis
   d. epistaxis

RS.47. Which respiratory condition in children and infants is characterized by obstruction of the larynx, hoarseness, and a barking cough?
   a. asthma
   b. croup
   c. diphtheria
   d. pneumonia

RS.48. Which term means a neoplasm composed of immature undifferentiated cells?
   a. adenocarcinoma
   b. blastoma
   c. malignant melanoma
   d. squamous cell carcinoma

RS.49.   Which of these sexually transmitted diseases is caused by a spirochete?

    a. chlamydia

    b. gonorrhea

    c. syphilis

    d. trichomonas

RS.50.   Which term describes a blood clot attached to the interior wall of a vein or artery?

    a. embolism

    b. embolus

    c. thrombosis

    d. thrombus

SENTENCE COMPLETION

Write the *answer*, spelled correctly, on the line provided.

RS.51. The term meaning abnormal enlargement of the liver is _____.

RS.52. The term meaning a pounding or racing heart is _____.

RS.53. The surgical removal of a portion of the tissue surrounding the heart is a/an

_____.

RS.54. A surgical connection between two hollow or tubular structures is a/an _____.

RS.55. Medication administered to expand the opening of the passages into the lungs is a/an

_____.

TRUE/FALSE

If the statement is true, write **T** on the line. If the statement is false, write **F** on the line.

RS.56. _____ Ileus is a temporary stoppage of intestinal peristalsis.

RS.57. _____ Hypothyroidism is a condition of excessive thyroid hormones in the blood.

RS.58. _____ Hysterorrhexis means to suture the uterus.

RS.59. _____ Nyctalopia is also known as night blindness.

RS.60. _____ Hypoglycemia is an abnormally low concentration of glucose in the blood.

RS.61. _____ Volvulus is the telescoping of one part of the intestine into the opening of an immediately adjacent part.

RS.62. _____ Nocturia is excessive urination during the night.

RS.63. _____ Myelography is a radiographic study of the bone marrow after the injection of a contrast medium.

RS.64. _____ Muscular dystrophy is a group of inherited muscle disorders that cause muscle weakness without affecting the nervous system.

RS.65. _____ Nephromalacia is abnormal hardening of the kidney.

CLINICAL CONDITIONS

Write the *term*, spelled correctly, on the line provided.

RS.66. Jewel Martin has a progressive autoimmune disorder characterized by scattered patches of demyelination of nerve fibers of the brain and spinal cord. The medical term for this condition is

_____ _____.

RS.67. Mr. Kuebler suffers from fine muscle tremors, has a masklike facial expression, and walks with a shuffling gait. The medical term for his progressive condition is _____

_____.

RS.68. José Ramirez told his friends that he had a heart attack. The medical term for this is a/an
_____ _____.

RS.69. Wayne Oliveri, who works all day at a keyboard, was diagnosed as having inflammation of the tendons passing through the carpal tunnel of the wrist. The condition is known as
_____ _____ syndrome.

RS.70. After an accident, Todd suffered from nerve pain caused by pressure on the spinal nerve roots in the neck region. The medical term for this condition is _____
_____.

RS.71. Nurse Ortega observed his patient's pattern of alternating periods of rapid breathing, slow breathing, and the absence of breathing. He recorded this on the chart as _____
_____ respiration.

RS.72. At age 45, George was diagnosed as having a hereditary disorder with symptoms that first appear in midlife and cause the irreversible and progressive loss of muscle control and mental ability. George has
_____ disease.

RS.73. Megan Wilson's surgeon removed her gallbladder while working through very small openings in the abdominal wall. The medical term for this procedure is a/an _____
_____.

RS.74. Rashondra is abnormally afraid of being in narrow or enclosed spaces. This medical term for this condition is _____.

RS.75. Brian was diagnosed as having peptic ulcers in the upper part of the small intestine. The medical term for this condition is _____ _____.

WHICH IS THE CORRECT MEDICAL TERM?

Circle the *letter* of the correct answer.

RS.76. Which term means the removal or destruction of the function of a body part?

   a. ablation

   b. abrasion

   c. cryosurgery

   d. exfoliative cytology

RS.77. Which term means a woman who has delivered one child?

   a. nulligravida

   b. nullipara

   c. primigravida

   d. primipara

RS.78. Which term means inflammation of the pancreas?

   a. pancreatalgia

   b. pancreatectomy

   c. pancreatitis

   d. pancreatotomy

RS.79. Which term means an abnormally increased amount of cerebrospinal fluid within the brain?

   a. hydrocele

   b. hydrocephalus

   c. hydronephrosis

   d. hydroureter

RS.80.   Which term means the surgical repair of the vagina?
   a. colpopexy
   b. colporrhaphy
   c. vaginoplasty
   d. valvoplasty

WORD BUILDING WITH THE "DOUBLE RR'S"

Write the *term*, spelled correctly, on the line provided.

RS.81. The term meaning to suture torn fascia is _____.

RS.82. The term meaning an excessive flow of mucus from the nose is _____.

RS.83. The term meaning rupture of the bladder is _____.

RS.84. The term meaning rupture of the stomach is _____.

RS.85. The term meaning bleeding from the spleen is _____.

RS.86. The term meaning to suture the ends of a severed nerve is _____.

RS.87. The term meaning bleeding from the ureter is _____.

RS.88. The term meaning the rupture of a muscle is _____.

RS.89. The term meaning the excessive flow of gastric secretions is _____.

RS.90. The term meaning to suture the tissue surrounding the heart is _____.

MEDICAL SPECIALTY REVIEW

Write the *term*, spelled correctly, on the line provided.

RS.91. A specialist in diagnosing and treating diseases, disorders, and problems associated with aging is a/an
   _____.

RS.92. A specialist, other than a physician, trained in administering anesthesia is a/an
   _____.

RS.93. A specialist in measuring the accuracy of vision to determine if corrective lenses or eyeglasses are needed is
   a/an _____.

RS.94. A specialist in diagnosing and treating diseases and disorders of the female reproductive system is a/an
   _____.

RS.95. A specialist in diagnosing, treating, and preventing disorders and diseases of children is a/an
   _____.

RS.96. A specialist in manipulative treatment of disorders originating from misalignment of the spine is a/an
   _____.

RS.97. A specialist in the prevention and treatment of disorders of the tissues surrounding the teeth is a/an
   _____.

RS.98. A specialist in diagnosing and treating diseases and disorders of the lungs and associated tissues is a/an
   _____.

RS.99. A specialist in diagnosing, treating, and correcting disorders of the foot is a/an
   _____.

RS.100. A specialist in providing medical care to women during pregnancy, childbirth, and immediately thereafter
   is a/an _____.

CONFIRMING MASTERY: SIMULATED MEDICAL TERMINOLOGY FINAL TEST

Grade _____ Name _____

Circle the *letter* of the correct answer.

FT.1.   Which medical term describes a torn or ragged wound?

    a. fissure

    b. fistula

    c. laceration

    d. lesion

FT.2.   The term cystopexy means

    a. drooping of the urinary bladder.

    b. inflammation of the gallbladder.

    c. laparoscopic examination of the gallbladder.

    d. surgical fixation of the urinary bladder.

FT.3.   Which medical term is commonly known as a heart attack?

    a. arthrostenosis

    b. myocardial infarction

    c. transient ischemic attack

    d. ventricular fibrillation

FT.4.   Which term means inflammation of the connective tissues that enclose the spinal cord and brain?

    a. encephalitis

    b. encephalopathy

    c. meningitis

    d. myelopathy

FT.5.   Which disease is also known as osteitis deformans?

    a. Crohn's disease

    b. Ewing's sarcoma

    c. Paget's disease

    d. Raynaud's phenomenon

FT.6.   The term myorrhexis means

    a. bleeding from the spinal cord.

    b. rupture of a muscle.

    c. rupture of the spinal cord.

    d. to suture a muscle.

FT.7.   Which term means abnormal softening of the kidney?

    a. nephromalacia

    b. nephrosclerosis

    c. neuromalacia

    d. neurosclerosis

FT.8.   A life-threatening complication of uncontrolled diabetes mellitus is

    a. an embolism.

    b. a thrombus.

    c. convulsions.

    d. diabetic ketoacidosis.

FT.9.   A carotid endarterectomy is performed to

    a. prevent a heart attack.

    b. prevent a stroke.

    c. relieve angina symptoms.

    d. treat hypertension.

FT.10. Which medical term means the flow of pus from the ear?

    a. otopyorrhea

    b. otorrhagia

    c. pyoderma

    d. pyosalpinx

FT.11. Which term is commonly known as itching?

    a. perfusion

    b. pruritus

    c. purpura

    d. suppuration

FT.12. Which term means spasmodic choking pain due to interference with the oxygen supply to the heart muscle?

    a. angina pectoris

    b. claudication

    c. cyanosis

    d. myocardial infarction

FT.13. Which condition is also known as trigeminal neuralgia?

    a. Hodgkin's disease

    b. Lou Gehrig's disease

    c. tic douloureux

    d. spasmodic torticollis

FT.14. Which term means an unexpected reaction to a drug?

    a. adverse

    b. idiosyncratic

c. placebo

d. palliative

FT.15. Which term means a prediction of the probable course and outcome of a disease or disorder?

a. differential diagnosis

b. diagnosis

c. prognosis

d. syndrome

FT.16. Which term means blue discoloration of the skin caused by a lack of adequate oxygen?

a. cyanosis

b. erythroderma

c. leukoplakia

d. melanosis

FT.17. A Colles' fracture is associated with which bone disease?

a. osteomalacia

b. osteomyelitis

c. osteoporosis

d. otosclerosis

FT.18. Which medical term is commonly known as bed-wetting?

a. nocturnal myoclonus

b. nocturnal enuresis

c. nocturia

d. urinary incontinence

FT.19. Which medical term describes any benign skin condition in which there is overgrowth and thickening of the epidermis?

a. epithelioma

b. keratosis

c. melanoma

d. papilloma

FT.20. Which term means inflammation of the lymph nodes?

a. adenoiditis

b. angiitis

c. lymphadenitis

d. lymphangioma

FT.21. Which term describes a sudden, involuntary contraction of a muscle?

a. adhesion

b. contracture

c. spasm

d. stricture

FT.22. Which respiratory disease is commonly known as whooping cough?

a. croup

b. diphtheria

c. emphysema

d. pertussis

FT.23. Which body system is affected by the autoimmune disorder known as Crohn's disease?

a. digestive

b. endocrine

c. nervous

d. reproductive

FT.24. Which condition is commonly known as low back pain?

a. kyphosis

b. lordosis

c. lumbago

d. scoliosis

FT.25. Which term means the surgical creation of an opening between the small intestine and the body surface?

a. colostomy

b. enteropexy

c. gastroptosis

d. ileostomy

FT.26. Which visualization technique is used to examine body parts in motion?

a. computed tomography

b. fluoroscopy

c. magnetic resonance imaging

d. radiography

FT.27. Which term means bleeding from the pharynx?

a. epistaxis

b. pharyngoplegia

c. pharyngorrhagia

d. pharyngorrhea

FT.28. Which autoimmune disease gradually destroys thyroid tissue?

a. Cushing's syndrome

b. goiter

c. Hashimoto's

d. Parkinson's disease

FT.29. Which term means a pus-producing inflammation of the uterus?

a. leukorrhea

b. metrorrhea

    c. pyometritis

    d. pyosalpinx

FT.30. Which term describes the syndrome characterized by sudden, severe, sharp headache usually present only on one side?

    a. cephalagia

    b. migraine headache

    c. myxedema

    d. tic douloureux

FT.31. Which term means vomiting blood?

    a. epistaxis

    b. hemarthrosis

    c. hematemesis

    d. hyperemesis

FT.32. Which term describes the condition commonly known as a bruise?

    a. ecchymosis

    b. exophthalmos

    c. hematoma

    d. hemangioma

FT.33. Which term means abnormally rapid, deep breathing resulting in decreased levels of carbon dioxide at the cellular level?

    a. apnea

    b. dyspnea

    c. hyperventilation

    d. hypoventilation

FT.34. Which medical term means difficult or painful urination?

    a. dyskinesia

    b. dyspepsia

    c. dysphagia

    d. dysuria

FT.35. Which term means a false personal belief that is maintained despite obvious proof to the contrary?

    a. delirium

    b. delusion

    c. dementia

    d. hallucination

FT.36. Which type of abnormal heartbeat is known as tachycardia?

    a. fast

    b. fluttering

    c. weak

    d. slow

FT.37. Which eye condition is characterized by increased intraocular pressure?
  a. cataracts
  b. glaucoma
  c. macular degeneration
  d. monochromatism

FT.38. Which diagnostic tool is used to image the brain and spinal cord?
  a. echoencephalography
  b. electroencephalography
  c. magnetic resonance imaging
  d. ultrasound

FT.39. Which vision condition is commonly known as nearsightedness?
  a. hyperopia
  b. myopia
  c. presbyopia
  d. strabismus

FT.40. Which body cavity protects the brain?
  a. anterior
  b. cranial
  c. superior
  d. ventral

FT.41. Which term means a hernia of the bladder through the vaginal wall?
  a. cystocele
  b. cystopexy
  c. vaginocele
  d. vesicovaginal fissure

FT.42. Which term means a violent shaking up or jarring of the brain caused by a direct blow or explosion?
  a. cerebral concussion
  b. cerebral contusion
  c. intracerebral hematoma
  d. subdural hematoma

FT.43. Which term means a ringing sound in the ears?
  a. presbycusis
  b. syncope
  c. tinnitus
  d. vertigo

FT.44. Which term means a sudden and widespread outbreak of a disease within a population group or area?
  a. endemic
  b. epidemic

    c. pandemic

    d. syndrome

FT.45. Which term means an excessive flow of gastric secretions?

    a. achlorhydria

    b. aerophagia

    c. gastrorrhea

    d. gastrorrhexis

FT.46. Which term describes a small, flat, discolored lesion such as a freckle?

    a. macule

    b. papule

    c. plaque

    d. vesicle

FT.47. The Western blot blood test is used to

    a. confirm an HIV infection.

    b. detect hepatitis B.

    c. diagnose Kaposi's sarcoma.

    d. test for tuberculosis.

FT.48. Which term means excessive uterine bleeding occurring both during the menses and at irregular intervals?

    a. dysmenorrhea

    b. menometrorrhagia

    c. menorrhagia

    d. mittelschmerz

FT.49. Which term describes an injury that does not break the skin and is characterized by swelling, discoloration, and pain?

    a. concussion

    b. contusion

    c. laceration

    d. lesion

FT.50. Which term describes an abnormal rattle or crackle-like respiratory sound heard during inspiration?

    a. bruit

    b. rale

    c. rhonchus

    d. stridor

FT.51. Which medical term is commonly known as wear-and-tear arthritis?

    a. gouty arthritis

    b. osteoarthritis

    c. rheumatoid arthritis

    d. spondylosis

FT.52. Which term means to free a tendon from adhesions?

    a. tenodesis

    b. tenolysis

    c. tenorrhaphy

    d. tenotomy

FT.53. The term debilitated means

    a. lacking adequate fluid.

    b. mental impairment.

    c. mentally confused due to a high fever.

    d. weakened or having lost strength.

FT.54. Which term describes a progressive degenerative disease characterized by disturbance of structure and function of the liver?

    a. cirrhosis

    b. hepatitis A

    c. hepatitis E

    d. jaundice

FT.55. Which procedure removes waste products directly from the blood of patients whose kidneys no longer function?

    a. diuresis

    b. epispadias

    c. hemodialysis

    d. peritoneal dialysis

FT.56. Which medical condition is commonly known as fainting?

    a. comatose

    b. narcolepsy

    c. stupor

    d. syncope

FT.57. Which term means a deficiency of blood supply due to the constriction or obstruction of a blood vessel?

    a. embolism

    b. infarction

    c. ischemia

    d. thrombosis

FT.58. Which term means an accumulation of blood in the pleural cavity?

    a. hemophilia

    b. hemoptysis

    c. hemostasis

    d. hemothorax

FT.59. Which term means the return of swallowed food into the mouth?

    a. emesis

    b. nausea

    c. reflux

    d. regurgitation

FT.60. Which condition is caused by prolonged exposure to high levels of cortisol?

    a. Addison's disease

    b. Cushing's syndrome

    c. Huntington's disease

    d. Parkinson's disease

FT.61. Which term describes a yellow discoloration of the skin caused by abnormal amounts of bilirubin in the blood?

    a. cyanosis

    b. ileus

    c. jaundice

    d. volvulus

FT.62. Which term means excessive urination?

    a. anuria

    b. oliguria

    c. polyuria

    d. pyuria

FT.63. Which term means the surgical removal of the gallbladder?

    a. cholecystectomy

    b. cholecystostomy

    c. cholecystotomy

    d. choledocholithotomy

FT.64. Which blood test is used to detect the presence of inflammation in the body?

    a. agglutination

    b. a platelet count

    c. complete blood cell count

    d. erythrocyte sedimentation rate

FT.65. Which term means a closed sac or pouch containing fluid or semisolid material?

    a. abscess

    b. cyst

    c. pustule

    d. ulcer

FT.66. Which type of injection is administered within the substance of a muscle?

    a. intradermal

    b. intramuscular

    c. intravenous

    d. subcutaneous

FT.67. Which term means abnormal tipping forward of the uterus and cervix?

  a. anteversion

  b. prolapse

  c. retroflexion

  d. retroversion

FT.68. Which term means inflammation of the brain?

  a. encephalitis

  b. mastitis

  c. meningitis

  d. myelitis

FT.69. Which term means a spasm or twitching of a muscle or group of muscles?

  a. contractures

  b. myoclonus

  c. seizures

  d. tremors

FT.70. Which term describes the condition when the heart is unable to pump enough blood to meet the body's needs?

  a. congestive heart failure

  b. hypoperfusion

  c. myocarditis

  d. mitral valve prolapse

FT.71. Which term means a hospital-acquired infection?

  a. functional disorder

  b. iatrogenic illness

  c. idiopathic disorder

  d. nosocomial infection

FT.72. Which term means a malignant tumor that arises from connective tissue?

  a. blastoma

  b. carcinoma

  c. malignant melanoma

  d. sarcoma

FT.73. Which term describes the eye disorder that may develop as a complication of diabetes?

  a. diabetic neuropathy

  b. diabetic retinopathy

  c. papilledema

  d. retinal detachment

FT.74. Which term describes an eating disorder characterized by refusing to maintain a minimally normal body weight and an intense fear of gaining weight?

  a. anorexia nervosa

  b. bulimia nervosa

c. hypochondriasis

d. pica

FT.75. Which term means the presence of blood in the urine?

   a. albuminuria

   b. blood urea nitrogen

   c. hematuria

   d. proteinuria

FT.76. Which term describes the condition caused when a blood vessel in the brain leaks or ruptures?

   a. cerebral hematoma

   b. embolism

   c. hemorrhagic stroke

   d. ischemic stroke

FT.77. Which term describes the condition characterized by enlargement of the hands and feet caused by excessive secretion of the growth hormone *after* puberty?

   a. acromegaly

   b. acrophobia

   c. cretinism

   d. gigantism

FT.78. Which terms means an ingrown toenail?

   a. cryptorchidism

   b. onychocryptosis

   c. onychophagia

   d. oophoropexy

FT.79. An otoscope is used to examine the

   a. adnexa of the eye.

   b. auditory canal and tympanic membrane.

   c. eustachian tube.

   d. retina and optic nerve of the eye.

FT.80. Which term means protrusion of part of the stomach through the esophageal opening in the diaphragm?

   a. esophageal hernia

   b. esophageal varices

   c. hiatal hernia

   d. hiatal varices

FT.81. Which term means a surgical incision of the vulva to facilitate delivery of a baby?

   a. episiorrhaphy

   b. episiotomy

   c. epispadias

   d. epistaxis

FT.82.   Which term describes a condition of severe itching of the external female genitalia?

    a. colpitis

    b. leukorrhea

    c. pruritus vulvae

    d. vaginal candidiasis

FT.83.   Which term describes an infestation commonly known as head lice?

    a. pediculosis capitis

    b. pediculosis pubis

    c. tinea capitis

    d. tinea pedis

FT.84.   Which instrument is used to enlarge the opening of a canal or body cavity to make it possible to inspect its interior?

    a. endoscope

    b. speculum

    c. sphygmomanometer

    d. stethoscope

FT.85.   Cellulitis is a

    a. diffuse infection of connective tissue.

    b. dry patch made up of excess dead epidermal cells.

    c. groove or crack-like sore.

    d. localized collection of pus.

FT.86.   Which term means a malignant tumor composed of cells derived from hemopoietic tissues of the bone marrow?

    a. mycosis

    b. myelitis

    c. myeloma

    d. myelosis

FT.87.   Which term means an inflammation of the lungs in which the air sacs fill with pus and other liquid?

    a. pneumoconiosis

    b. pneumonia

    c. pneumonitis

    d. pneumothorax

FT.88.   Which term means ankylosis of the bones of the middle ear resulting in a conductive hearing loss?

    a. labyrinthitis

    b. mastoiditis

    c. osteosclerosis

    d. otosclerosis

FT.89.   Which term means to free a tendon from adhesions?

    a. arthrodesis

    b. arthrolysis

c. tenodesis

d. tenolysis

FT.90.   Which term means to suture the vagina?

a. colporrhaphy

b. cystorrhaphy

c. hepatorrhaphy

d. hysterorrhaphy

FT.91.   Which term means the surgical removal of plaque from the interior lining of an artery?

a. angiectomy

b. arteriectomy

c. atherectomy

d. arthrectomy

FT.92.   Which term means abnormally increased motor function or activity?

a. bradykinesia

b. dyskinesia

c. hyperkinesia

d. hypokinesia

FT.93.   Which term means difficulty in swallowing?

a. dyspepsia

b. dysphagia

c. dysphonia

d. dysplasia

FT.94.   Which term means the process of recording electrical brain wave activity?

a. echoencephalography

b. electroencephalography

c. electromyography

d. electroneuromyography

FT.95.   Which term means a woman who has never been pregnant?

a. nulligravida

b. nullipara

c. primigravida

d. primipara

FT.96.   Which eye condition causes the loss of central vision but not total blindness?

a. cataracts

b. glaucoma

c. macular degeneration

d. presbyopia

FT.97. Which term means the surgical removal of excess skin for the elimination of wrinkles?
   a. blepharoplasty
   b. plication
   c. rhytidectomy
   d. sclerotherapy

FT.98. Which term means a group of inherited muscle disorders that cause muscle weakness without affecting the nervous system?
   a. multiple sclerosis
   b. muscular dystrophy
   c. myasthenia gravis
   d. Parkinson's disease

FT.99. Which term describes the process by which cancer spreads from one place to another?
   a. metabolism
   b. metastasis
   c. metastasize
   d. staging

FT.100. Which term means a collection of blood trapped within tissues?
   a. hemangioma
   b. hematemesis
   c. hematoma
   d. hematuria

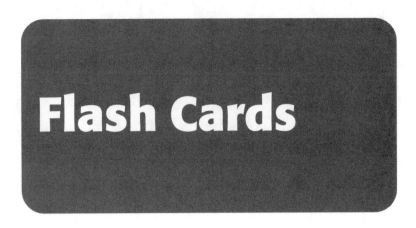

Flash Cards

INSTRUCTIONS

- Carefully remove the flash card pages from the workbook and cut them apart to create 160 flash cards.
- There are three types of cards: **prefixes** (such as *a-* and *hyper-),* **suffixes** (such as *-graphy* and *-rrhagia*), and **word roots/combining forms** (such as *gastr/o* and *arthr/o*). For the prefixes and suffixes, the type of word part is listed on the front on each card. The definition is on the back.
- The word root/combining form cards are arranged by body system. This allows you to sort out the cards you want to study based on where you are in the book. Use the "general" cards as they apply throughout your course.
- Use the flash cards to memorize word parts, to test yourself, and as a periodic review.
- By putting cards together, you can create terms just as you did in the challenge word building exercises.

WORD PART GAMES

Here are games you can play with one or more partners to help you learn word parts using your flash cards.

THE REVIEW GAME

Word Parts Up: Shuffle the deck of flash cards. Put the pile, *word parts up*, in the center of the desk. Take turns choosing a card from anywhere in the deck and giving the definition of the word part shown. If you get it right, you get to keep it. If you miss, it goes into the discard pile. When the draw pile is gone, whoever has the largest pile wins.

Definitions Up: Shuffle the deck of flash cards and place them with the *definition side up*. Play the review game the same way.

THE CREATE-A-WORD GAME

Shuffle the deck and deal each person 14 cards, *word parts up*. Place the remaining draw pile in the center of the desk, *word parts down*.

Each player should try to create as many legitimate medical words as possible using the cards he or she has been dealt. Then take turns discarding one card (word part up, in the discard pile) and taking one. When it is your turn to discard a card, you may choose either the card the previous player discarded, or a "mystery card" from the draw pile. Continue working on words until all the cards in the draw pile have been taken.

To score, each player must define every word created correctly. If the definition is correct, the player receives one point for each card used. If it is incorrect, two points are deducted for each card in that word. Cards left unused each count as one point off. Whoever has the highest number of points wins. *Note:* Use your medical dictionary if there is any doubt that a word is legitimate!

kidney

retina

renal pelvis, bowl of kidney

sclera, white of eye, hard

kidney

tympanic membrane, eardrum

ureter

urinary bladder, cyst, sac of fluid

urethra

stone, calculus

Special Senses

RETIN/O

Urinary System

NEPHR/O

ecial Senses and Integumentary System

SCLER/O

Urinary System

PYEL/O

Special Senses

TYMPAN/O

Urinary System

REN/O

Urinary System

CYST/O

Urinary System

URETER/O

Urinary System

LITH/O

Urinary System

URETHR/O

chest	rib
horny, hard, cornea	skull
tympanic membrane, eardrum	spinal cord, bone marrow
eye, vision	bone
ear, hearing	vertebrae, vertebral column, back bone

Skeletal System

COST/O

Skeletal and Respiratory Systems

THORAC/O

Skeletal System

CRANI/O

Special Senses and Integumentary System

KERAT/O

Skeletal System

MYEL/O

Special Senses

MYRING/O

Skeletal System

OSS/E, OSS/I, OST/O, OSTE/O

Special Senses

OPTIC/O, OPT/O

Skeletal System

Special Senses

OT/O

SPONDYL/O

lung	bronchial tube, bronchus
trachea, windpipe	larynx, voice box
crooked, bent, stiff	throat, pharynx
joint	pleura, side of the body
cartilage	lung, air

Respiratory System

BRONCH/O, BRONCHI/O

Respiratory System

PULM/O, PULMON/O

Respiratory System

LARYNG/O

Respiratory System

TRACHE/O

Respiratory System

PHARYNG/O

Skeletal System

ANKLY/O

Respiratory System

PLEUR/O

Skeletal System

ARTHR/O

Respiratory System

PNEUM/O, PNEUMON/O

Skeletal System

CHONDR/O

ovary

vagina

testicles, testis, testes

uterus

uterine (fallopian) tube, auditory
(eustachian) tube

menstruation, menses

uterus

uterus

vagina

egg

Reproductive Systems

COLP/O

Reproductive Systems

OOPHOR/O, OVARI/O

Reproductive Systems

HYSTER/O

Reproductive Systems

ORCH/O, ORCHI/O, ORCHID/O

Reproductive Systems

MEN/O

Reproductive Systems and Special Senses

SALPING/O

Reproductive Systems

METR/O, METRI/O

Reproductive Systems

UTER/O

Reproductive Systems

OO/O, OV/I, OV/O

Reproductive Systems

VAGIN/O

muscle

nail

tendon, stretch out, extend, strain

dry

brain

gland

meninges, membranes

spleen

nerve, nerve tissue

fascia, fibrous band

Integumentary System	Muscular System
UNGU/O	**MY/O**

Integumentary System	Muscular System
XER/O	**TEN/O, TEND/O, TENDIN/O**

Lymphatic System	Nervous System
ADEN/O	**ENCEPHAL/O**

Lymphatic System	Nervous System
SPLEN/O	**MENING/O**

Muscular System	Nervous System
FASCI/O	**NEUR/I, NEUR/O**

tumor	disease, suffering, feeling, emotion
skin	pus
skin	fever, fire
sweat	flesh (connective tissue)
sebum	cancerous

General	Immune System
PATH/O	**ONC/O**

General	Integumentary System
PY/O	**CUTANE/O**

General	Integumentary System
PYR/O	**DERM/O, DERMAT/O**

General	Integumentary System
SARC/O	**HIDR/O**

Immune System	Integumentary System
CARCIN/O	**SEB/O**

abdomen, abdominal wall	coronary, crown
white	blue
fat, lipid	cell
black, dark	red
fungus	tissue

General

CORON/O

General

LAPAR/O

General

CYAN/O

General

LEUK/O

General

CYT/O

General

LIP/O

General

ERYTHR/O

General

MELAN/O

General

HIST/O

General

MYC/O

thyroid gland	liver
fat	sigmoid colon
white	adrenal glands
head	sex gland
neck, cervix (neck of uterus)	pancreas

Digestive System

HEPAT/O

Endocrine System

THYR/O, THYROID/O

Digestive System

SIGMOID/O

General

ADIP/O

Endocrine System

ADREN/O, ADRENAL/O

General

ALBIN/O

crine and Reproductive Systems

GONAD/O

General

CEPHAL/O

ndocrine and Digestive Systems

PANCREAT/O

General

CERVIC/O

colon, large intestine	clot
duodenum	vein
small intestine	sound
esophagus	radiation, x-rays
stomach	gallbladder

Cardiovascular System	Digestive System
THROMB/O	**COL/O, COLON/O**
Cardiovascular System	Digestive System
VEN/O	**DUODEN/I, DUODEN/O**
Diagnostic Procedures	Digestive System
ECH/O	**ENTER/O**
Diagnostic Procedures	Digestive System
RADI/O	**ESOPHAG/O**
Digestive System	Digestive System
CHOLECYST/O	**GASTR/O**

artery	abnormal narrowing
plaque, fatty substance	to crush
heart	urination, urine
blood, pertaining to the blood	pertaining to blood or lymph vessels
vein	aorta

-STENOSIS

ARTER/O, ARTERI/O

-TRIPSY

ATHER/O

-URIA

CARD/O, CARDI/O

ANGI/O

HEM/O, HEMAT/O

AORT/O

PHLEB/O

suffix

-OLOGIST

suffix

-OTOMY

suffix

-OLOGY

suffix

-PATHY

suffix

-OMA

suffix

-PAUSE

suffix

-OSIS

suffix

-PEXY

suffix

-OSTOMY

suffix

-PLASTY

surgical incision

specialist

disease, suffering, feeling, emotion

the science or study of

stopping

tumor

surgical fixation, to put in place

abnormal condition

surgical repair

surgical creation of an opening

suffix

-PLEGIA

suffix

-RRHEA

suffix

-PNEA

suffix

-RRHEXIS

suffix

-PTOSIS

suffix

-SCLEROSIS

suffix

-RRHAGIA, -RRHAGE

suffix

-SCOPE

suffix

-RRHAPHY

suffix

-SCOPY

abnormal flow or discharge

paralysis

rupture

breathing

abnormal hardening

prolapse, drooping forward

instrument for visual examination

bleeding, abnormal excessive fluid disc

to see, visual examination

to suture

inflammation

sensation, feeling

breakdown, separation, setting free,
destruction, loosening

record

abnormal softening

process of recording

enlargement

state or condition

tissue death

pertaining to

suffix

-ESTHESIA

suffix

-ITIS

suffix

-GRAM, -GRAPH

suffix

-LYSIS

suffix

-GRAPHY

suffix

-MALACIA

suffix

-IA

suffix

-MEGALY

suffix

-IC

suffix

-NECROSIS

cell

pertaining to, relating to

surgical fixation of bone or joint, to bind, tie together

pain, suffering

surgical removal

pertaining to

stretching, enlargement

hernia, tumor, swelling

blood, blood condition

surgical puncture to remove fluid

suffix

-AC, -AL

suffix

-CYTE

suffix

-ALGIA

suffix

-DESIS

suffix

-ARY

suffix

-ECTOMY

suffix

-CELE

suffix

-ECTASIS

suffix

-CENTESIS

suffix

-EMIA

after	within, inside
before	new, strange
below	excessive, through
above, excessive	surrounding, around
fast, rapid	many

prefix

INTRA-

prefix

POST-

prefix

NEO-

prefix

PRE-

prefix

PER-

prefix

SUB-

prefix

PERI-

prefix

SUPER-, SUPRA-

prefix

POLY-

prefix

TACHY-

within, in, inside	without, away from, negative, not
half	before, toward
excessive, increased	against, counter
deficient, decreased	slow
between, among	bad, difficult, painful

prefix

A-, AN-

prefix

END-, ENDO-

prefix

ANTE-

prefix

HEMI-

prefix

ANTI-

prefix

HYPER-

prefix

BRADY-

prefix

HYPO-

prefix

DYS-

prefix

INTER-